BASICS OF BALANCED DIET

Ifeanyichukwu Ezekwem

CONTENTS

Title Page

Introduction To Balanced Diet   2

Nutrients And Their Roles   10

Calorie Needs Of Different Individuals   20

Portion Control   28

Food Groups   36

Hydration And Its Importance   45

Balancing Macronutrients   55

Fiber And Whole Grains, Sugars And Added Sugars, Healthy Fats, Micreonutrients   62

Meal Planning   74

Dietary Guidelines   83

Special Dies For Special Classes Of People   92

Sustainable Eating   102

About The Author   114

Book Overview

The book "Basics of Balanced Diet" provides a comprehensive overview of the principles and importance of maintaining a balanced diet. In this book, readers will gain a clear understanding of the role of nutrients and their impact on overall health and well-being. The book explores the concept of calorie needs for different individuals and emphasizes the significance of portion control in maintaining a healthy weight.

Furthermore, "Basics of Balanced Diet" delves into the various food groups and their contributions to a well-rounded diet. The book highlights the importance of hydration and its impact on bodily functions. It also provides insights into the balancing of macronutrients, such as carbohydrates, proteins, and fats, to optimize nutrition. Additionally, the book emphasizes the significance of incorporating fiber and whole grains into one's diet, while also addressing the potential risks associated with sugars and added sugars.

Moreover, "Basics of Balanced Diet" sheds light on the importance of consuming healthy fats and the role of micronutrients in supporting overall health. The book offers practical guidance on meal planning and explores dietary guidelines that can serve as a foundation for a balanced diet. It also provides insights into special diets tailored for specific classes of people, such as athletes, pregnant women, and individuals with certain medical conditions. Lastly, the book touches upon the concept of sustainable eating and its impact on personal health and the environment.

INTRODUCTION TO BALANCED DIET

What is a Balanced Diet?

A balanced diet is a way of eating that provides all the essential nutrients, vitamins, and minerals that your body needs to function optimally. It involves consuming a variety of foods from different food groups in the right proportions to maintain good health and prevent nutritional deficiencies. A balanced diet is not about restricting or eliminating certain foods but rather about making informed choices and creating a healthy eating pattern.

To understand what a balanced diet entails, it is important to consider the different food groups and their respective contributions to our overall health. These food groups include fruits, vegetables, grains, protein sources, dairy products, and fats/oils. Each food group provides specific nutrients that are essential for our body's growth, development, and maintenance.

Fruits and vegetables are rich in vitamins, minerals, and antioxidants that help protect our bodies against diseases. They are also a great source of dietary fiber, which aids in digestion and helps maintain a healthy weight. Examples of fruits and vegetables include apples, oranges, spinach, broccoli, and carrots.

Grains, such as rice, bread, pasta, and cereals, are a significant source of carbohydrates, which provide energy for our daily activities. Whole grains, such as brown rice and whole wheat bread, are particularly beneficial as they contain more fiber and nutrients compared to refined grains.

Protein sources, such as lean meats, poultry, fish, beans, and legumes, are essential for building and repairing tissues, producing enzymes and hormones, and supporting a healthy immune system. Including a variety of protein sources in your diet ensures that you obtain all the essential amino acids your body needs.

Dairy products, such as milk, cheese, and yogurt, are rich in calcium, which is crucial for strong bones and teeth. They also provide protein and other essential nutrients. If you are lactose intolerant or follow a vegan diet, there are alternative sources of calcium, such as fortified plant-based milk and leafy green vegetables.

Fats and oils are necessary for our body to function properly, but it is important to choose healthy fats. Unsaturated fats, found in foods like avocados, nuts, and olive oil, are beneficial for heart health. On the other hand, saturated and trans fats, found in fried foods and processed snacks, should be limited as they can increase the risk of heart disease.

A balanced diet also involves consuming adequate amounts of water. Water is essential for hydration, digestion, nutrient absorption, temperature regulation, and overall bodily functions. It is recommended to drink at least 8 cups (64 ounces) of water per day, but individual needs may vary depending on factors such as activity level, climate, and overall health.

In addition to understanding the different food groups, portion control is another important aspect of a balanced diet. It is not only about what you eat but also how much you eat. Portion control helps prevent overeating and ensures that you are consuming the right amount of nutrients without exceeding your energy needs.

By following a balanced diet, you can reap numerous benefits for your overall health and well-being. It can help maintain a healthy weight, reduce the risk of chronic diseases such as heart disease, diabetes, and certain cancers, improve digestion, boost energy levels, enhance mood and mental clarity, and support a strong immune system.

In conclusion, a balanced diet is a way of eating that includes a variety of foods from different food groups in the right proportions. It provides all the essential nutrients, vitamins, and minerals that our bodies need to function optimally. By understanding the importance of each food group and practicing portion control, we can achieve and maintain good health. In the following sections, we will delve deeper into why a balanced diet is important, the benefits it offers, and common misconceptions surrounding it.

Why is a Balanced Diet Important?

A balanced diet is essential for maintaining good health and overall well-being. It provides the necessary nutrients, vitamins, and minerals that our bodies need to function properly. A diet that lacks balance can lead to various health issues and deficiencies, affecting our physical and mental health. In this section, we will explore the importance of a balanced diet and how it contributes to our overall health.

The Role of Nutrients

A balanced diet ensures that our bodies receive all the essential nutrients they need to perform their functions effectively. Nutrients can be broadly categorized into macronutrients and micronutrients. Macronutrients include carbohydrates, proteins, and fats, which provide energy and support various bodily functions. Micronutrients, on the other hand, include vitamins and minerals, which are required in smaller quantities but are equally important for maintaining optimal health.

Energy and Vitality

One of the primary reasons why a balanced diet is important is because it provides us with the energy we need to carry out our daily activities. Carbohydrates are the body's primary source of energy, and a balanced diet ensures an adequate intake of carbohydrates to fuel our activities. Proteins are essential for building and repairing tissues, while fats provide a concentrated source of energy and help in the absorption of fat-soluble vitamins.

When we consume a balanced diet, our bodies receive the necessary nutrients to function optimally, resulting in increased energy levels and overall vitality. This, in turn, allows us to perform better in our daily tasks, whether it's at work, school, or engaging in physical activities.

Disease Prevention

A balanced diet plays a crucial role in preventing various diseases and health conditions. Consuming a variety of fruits, vegetables, whole grains, lean proteins, and healthy fats provides our bodies with the necessary antioxidants, phytochemicals, and fiber that help boost our immune system and protect against chronic diseases such as heart disease, diabetes, and certain types of cancer.

For example, a diet rich in fruits and vegetables provides essential vitamins and minerals that support a healthy immune system, reducing the risk of infections and illnesses. Whole grains are a great source of dietary fiber, which aids in digestion and helps prevent conditions like constipation and diverticulosis. Including lean proteins in our diet helps build and repair tissues, supports a healthy metabolism, and keeps us feeling full and satisfied.

Weight Management

Maintaining a healthy weight is crucial for overall health and well-being. A balanced diet can help us achieve and maintain a healthy weight by providing the right balance of nutrients and controlling portion sizes. When we consume a diet that is high in nutrient-dense foods and low in processed and sugary foods, we are more likely to achieve a healthy weight and reduce the risk of obesity.

A balanced diet includes a variety of foods from different food groups, ensuring that we receive all the necessary nutrients while keeping our calorie intake in check. By focusing on whole, unprocessed foods and practicing portion control, we can maintain a healthy weight and reduce the risk of weight-related health issues such as diabetes, high blood pressure, and heart disease.

Mental Well-being

The importance of a balanced diet extends beyond physical health and also plays a significant role in our mental well-being. Research has shown that certain nutrients, such as omega-3 fatty acids found in fatty fish, and vitamins B6, B12, and folate found in leafy greens and legumes, can have a positive impact on our mood and mental health.

A diet lacking in essential nutrients can contribute to mood swings, fatigue, and even mental health disorders such as depression and anxiety. On the other hand, a balanced diet that includes a variety of nutrient-rich foods can help support brain health, improve cognitive function, and enhance overall mental well-being.

Longevity and Quality of Life

By adopting a balanced diet, we can significantly improve our chances of living a long and healthy life. A diet that is rich in nutrients and low in processed foods and unhealthy fats can help prevent chronic diseases, maintain a healthy weight, and support overall well-being.

Additionally, a balanced diet can also enhance the quality of life as we age. Proper nutrition plays a vital role in maintaining bone health, muscle strength, and cognitive function, which are all essential for maintaining independence and a high quality of life in older adults.

In conclusion, a balanced diet is of utmost importance for our overall health and well-being. It provides us with the necessary nutrients, energy, and protection against diseases. By adopting a balanced diet, we can enhance our physical and mental health, manage our weight effectively, and improve our chances of living a long and healthy life.

Benefits of a Balanced Diet

A balanced diet is not just about eating a variety of foods in the right proportions; it also offers numerous benefits for our overall health and well-being. When we provide our bodies with the essential nutrients it needs, we can experience a range of positive effects that can improve our quality of life. In this section, we will explore some of the key benefits of following a balanced diet.

1. Improved Energy Levels

One of the most noticeable benefits of a balanced diet is increased energy levels. When we consume a variety of nutrient-rich foods, our bodies receive the necessary fuel to function optimally. Carbohydrates, for example, are the body's primary source of energy, and including complex carbohydrates like whole grains, fruits, and vegetables in our diet can provide a steady release of energy throughout the day. Additionally, consuming adequate amounts of protein and healthy fats can help sustain energy levels and prevent energy crashes.

2. Enhanced Mental Clarity and Focus

A well-balanced diet not only nourishes our bodies but also supports our cognitive function. Certain nutrients, such as omega-3 fatty acids found in fatty fish, walnuts, and flaxseeds, have been linked to improved brain health and cognitive performance. Additionally, consuming a variety of fruits and vegetables rich in antioxidants can help protect brain cells from oxidative stress and promote mental clarity and focus. By fueling our brains with the right nutrients, we can enhance our ability to concentrate, think clearly, and maintain a positive mood.

3. Weight Management

Maintaining a healthy weight is crucial for overall well-being, and a balanced diet plays a significant role in weight management. By consuming a variety of nutrient-dense foods, we can feel satisfied and satiated while still meeting our nutritional needs. Whole foods, such as fruits, vegetables, lean proteins, and whole grains, are generally lower in calories and higher in fiber, which can help control hunger and prevent overeating. Additionally, a balanced diet can help regulate our metabolism, making it easier to achieve and maintain a healthy weight.

4. Stronger Immune System

A well-nourished body is better equipped to fight off infections and diseases. A balanced diet provides the essential vitamins, minerals, and antioxidants that support a robust immune system. For example, vitamin C, found in citrus fruits, berries, and leafy greens, is known for its immune-boosting properties. Similarly, zinc, found in lean meats, legumes, and nuts, plays a vital role in immune function. By incorporating a variety of nutrient-rich foods into our diet, we can strengthen our immune system and reduce the risk of falling ill.

5. Improved Digestive Health

A balanced diet that includes an adequate amount of fiber promotes good digestive health. Fiber helps regulate bowel movements, prevents constipation, and supports a healthy gut microbiome. Whole grains, fruits, vegetables, and legumes are excellent sources of dietary fiber. By including these foods in our diet, we can maintain a healthy digestive system, improve nutrient absorption, and reduce the risk of gastrointestinal disorders.

6. Reduced Risk of Chronic Diseases

Following a balanced diet has been associated with a lower risk of developing chronic diseases such as heart disease, diabetes, and certain types of cancer. A diet rich in fruits, vegetables, whole grains, lean proteins, and healthy fats provides the necessary nutrients and antioxidants that can help protect against these diseases. For example, a diet low in saturated and trans fats, found in processed foods and fatty meats, can help reduce the risk of heart disease. Similarly, consuming a variety of colorful fruits and vegetables can provide a range of antioxidants that may help prevent certain types of cancer.

7. Improved Sleep Quality

The foods we consume can significantly impact our sleep quality. A balanced diet that includes foods rich in tryptophan, such as turkey, chicken, nuts, and seeds, can promote the production of serotonin, a neurotransmitter that helps regulate sleep. Additionally, certain minerals like magnesium, found in leafy greens, nuts, and whole grains, can help relax the body and promote better sleep. By adopting a balanced diet, we can improve our sleep patterns, ensuring we wake up feeling refreshed and rejuvenated.

8. Enhanced Overall Well-being

Ultimately, following a balanced diet can lead to an improved overall sense of well-being. When we nourish our bodies with the right nutrients, we can experience increased vitality, improved mood, and a greater sense of self-confidence. A balanced diet can also positively impact our physical appearance, promoting healthy skin, hair, and nails. By prioritizing our nutritional needs, we can enhance our quality of life and enjoy the benefits of a healthier, happier self.

In conclusion, a balanced diet offers a multitude of benefits for our physical and mental well-being. From increased energy levels and improved cognitive function to weight management and reduced risk of chronic diseases, the advantages of following a balanced diet are undeniable. By making conscious choices to include a variety of nutrient-rich foods in our daily meals, we can reap the rewards of a healthier and more fulfilling life.

Common Misconceptions about Balanced Diet

A balanced diet is often misunderstood and surrounded by various misconceptions. These misconceptions can lead to confusion and prevent individuals from achieving optimal health and well-being. In this section, we will address some of the common misconceptions about a balanced diet and provide clarity on these topics.

Misconception 1: A Balanced Diet Means Restricting or Eliminating Certain Food Groups

One of the most prevalent misconceptions about a balanced diet is that it requires restricting or eliminating certain food groups. Some people believe that cutting out carbohydrates, fats, or even entire food groups like dairy or grains, is necessary for a healthy diet. However, this is not the case.

A balanced diet emphasizes the inclusion of all essential nutrients from various food groups. Each food group provides unique benefits and contributes to overall health. For example, carbohydrates are a primary source of energy, while proteins are essential for muscle repair and growth. Fats play a crucial role in hormone production and nutrient absorption. By eliminating or severely restricting any food group, you may miss out on vital nutrients, leading to imbalances in your diet.

Misconception 2: All Fats are Unhealthy

Another common misconception is that all fats are unhealthy and should be avoided. While it is true that certain types of fats, such as trans fats and saturated fats, can be detrimental to health when consumed in excess, not all fats are created equal.

Healthy fats, such as monounsaturated and polyunsaturated fats, are essential for the body's proper functioning. These fats can be found in foods like avocados, nuts, seeds, and fatty fish. They provide numerous health benefits, including supporting heart health, reducing inflammation, and aiding in the absorption of fat-soluble vitamins.

It is important to include these healthy fats in your diet in moderation and avoid excessive consumption of unhealthy fats. By understanding the difference between healthy and unhealthy fats, you can make informed choices and maintain a balanced diet.

Misconception 3: Skipping Meals Helps with Weight Loss

Many people believe that skipping meals, particularly breakfast, can aid in weight loss. However, this is a misconception that can have negative effects on your overall health and well-being.

Skipping meals, especially breakfast, can lead to increased hunger later in the day, causing you to overeat or make unhealthy food choices. Additionally, it can negatively impact your metabolism, making it harder for your body to burn calories efficiently.

Instead of skipping meals, focus on portion control and choosing nutrient-dense foods. Eating regular, balanced meals throughout the day can help stabilize blood sugar levels, maintain energy levels, and support healthy weight management.

Misconception 4: Supplements Can Replace a Balanced Diet

Supplements can be beneficial in certain situations, such as addressing specific nutrient deficiencies or supporting certain health conditions. However, they should not be seen as a replacement for a balanced diet.

Whole foods contain a wide range of nutrients, including vitamins, minerals, fiber, and phytochemicals, that work synergistically to support optimal health. While supplements can provide isolated nutrients, they lack the complex interactions found in whole foods.

It is always best to obtain nutrients from a variety of whole foods as part of a balanced diet. Supplements should be used under the guidance of a healthcare professional and should not be relied upon as the sole source of nutrition.

Misconception 5: A Balanced Diet is Expensive and Time-Consuming

Some individuals believe that maintaining a balanced diet is expensive and time-consuming. While it is true that healthy food choices can sometimes be more expensive, there are many ways to eat a balanced diet on a budget.

Planning meals, buying in bulk, and opting for seasonal produce can help reduce costs. Additionally, preparing meals at home allows you to have control over the ingredients and portion sizes, making it easier to maintain a balanced diet.

With proper planning and organization, it is possible to incorporate a balanced diet into a busy lifestyle. Simple strategies like meal prepping, batch cooking, and utilizing time-saving kitchen tools can help streamline the process and make healthy eating more accessible.

Misconception 6: A Balanced Diet is Bland and Boring

Some people believe that a balanced diet consists of tasteless and boring food options. However, this is far from the truth. A balanced diet can be both nutritious and delicious.

There are countless ways to add flavor and variety to your meals while still maintaining a balanced diet. Experimenting with herbs, spices, and different cooking techniques can transform simple ingredients into flavorful dishes. Additionally, incorporating a wide range of fruits, vegetables, whole grains, lean proteins, and healthy fats can provide a diverse and exciting array of flavors and textures.

By exploring different recipes, cuisines, and cooking methods, you can discover a world of delicious and nutritious options that align with a balanced diet.

Conclusion

Understanding and dispelling common misconceptions about a balanced diet is essential for achieving optimal health and well-being. By debunking these misconceptions, we can embrace the true principles of a balanced diet and make informed choices about our nutrition. Remember, a balanced diet is about moderation, variety, and nourishing your body with the nutrients it needs to thrive.

NUTRIENTS AND THEIR ROLES

Macronutrients

Macronutrients are the essential nutrients that our bodies require in large quantities to function properly. They provide us with energy, support growth and development, and help maintain overall health. The three main macronutrients are carbohydrates, proteins, and fats. Each macronutrient plays a unique role in the body and has specific functions and benefits.

Carbohydrates

Carbohydrates are the body's primary source of energy. They are found in a variety of foods, including grains, fruits, vegetables, and dairy products. Carbohydrates can be further classified into two types: simple carbohydrates and complex carbohydrates.

Simple carbohydrates, also known as sugars, are found in foods such as table sugar, honey, and fruit juices. They are quickly digested and provide a rapid source of energy. However, consuming excessive amounts of simple carbohydrates can lead to spikes in blood sugar levels and contribute to weight gain.

Complex carbohydrates, on the other hand, are found in foods like whole grains, legumes, and starchy vegetables. They are composed of long chains of sugar molecules and take longer to digest, providing a steady release of energy. Complex carbohydrates also contain fiber, which aids in digestion and helps maintain a feeling of fullness.

Including a variety of complex carbohydrates in your diet is important for sustained energy levels and overall health. Examples of healthy complex carbohydrates include whole wheat bread, brown rice, quinoa, oats, and sweet potatoes.

Proteins

Proteins are the building blocks of the body and are essential for growth, repair, and maintenance of tissues. They are made up of amino acids, which are linked together in various combinations. There are 20 different amino acids, and our bodies can produce some of them, while others must be obtained from the foods we eat.

Protein-rich foods include meat, poultry, fish, eggs, dairy products, legumes, and nuts. Animal-based proteins are considered complete proteins as they contain all the essential amino acids in the right proportions. Plant-based proteins, on the other hand, may lack one or more essential amino acids, but can be combined to form complete proteins.

Proteins play a vital role in many bodily functions, including the production of enzymes, hormones, and antibodies. They also help build and repair muscles, support immune function, and contribute to a feeling of satiety. Including a variety of protein sources in your diet ensures that you obtain all the essential amino acids your body needs.

Fats

Fats are often misunderstood and associated with weight gain and poor health. However, fats are an essential part of a balanced diet and play several important roles in the body. They provide a concentrated source of energy, help absorb fat-soluble vitamins, protect organs, and insulate the body.

There are different types of fats, including saturated fats, unsaturated fats, and trans fats. Saturated fats are primarily found in animal-based products such as meat, butter, and full-fat dairy. Consuming excessive amounts of saturated fats can increase the risk of heart disease and should be limited in the diet.

Unsaturated fats, on the other hand, are considered healthy fats and can be found in foods like avocados, nuts, seeds, and olive oil. They can help lower cholesterol levels and reduce the risk of heart disease when consumed in moderation.

Trans fats are artificial fats that are created through a process called hydrogenation. They are commonly found in processed foods, fried foods, and baked goods. Trans fats should be avoided as they have been linked to an increased risk of heart disease.

It is important to include a moderate amount of healthy fats in your diet to support overall health. Examples of healthy fats include avocados, nuts, seeds, olive oil, fatty fish like salmon and tuna, and natural nut butters.

Balancing Macronutrients

Achieving a balance of macronutrients is essential for optimal health and well-being. The specific ratio of macronutrients that works best for an individual can vary depending on factors such as age, sex, activity level, and overall health goals.

A balanced diet typically consists of approximately 45-65% of calories from carbohydrates, 10-35% from protein, and 20-35% from fats. However, it is important to note that these percentages can vary based on individual needs and preferences.

To achieve a balanced macronutrient intake, it is important to focus on consuming a variety of whole, unprocessed foods. This includes incorporating a mix of complex carbohydrates, lean proteins, and healthy fats into your meals and snacks.

For example, a balanced breakfast could include a bowl of oatmeal topped with fresh berries and a sprinkle of nuts or seeds. This provides a combination of complex carbohydrates, fiber, and healthy fats from the nuts or seeds. Adding a source of protein such as Greek yogurt or a boiled egg can further enhance the nutritional value of the meal.

Lunch and dinner can consist of a balance of lean proteins, whole grains, and vegetables. For instance, a grilled chicken breast served with quinoa and roasted vegetables provides a combination of protein, complex carbohydrates, and essential nutrients.

Snacks can also be balanced by combining a carbohydrate source with a protein or healthy fat. Examples include apple slices with almond butter, whole grain crackers with hummus, or a handful of nuts and dried fruit.

By focusing on a balanced macronutrient intake, you can ensure that your body receives the necessary nutrients for optimal health and function. It is important to listen to your body's needs and make adjustments as necessary to maintain a healthy balance.

Micronutrients

Micronutrients are essential nutrients that our bodies require in small amounts for proper functioning and overall health. Unlike macronutrients, which provide energy in the form of calories, micronutrients do not provide energy directly but play crucial roles in various physiological processes. Micronutrients include vitamins and minerals, which are necessary for the proper functioning of our immune system, metabolism, and overall well-being.

Vitamins

Vitamins are organic compounds that are essential for the normal growth, development, and maintenance of our bodies. They are classified into two categories: fat-soluble vitamins (A, D, E, and K) and water-soluble vitamins (B vitamins and vitamin C).

Fat-Soluble Vitamins

Vitamin A: This vitamin is important for maintaining healthy vision, promoting proper immune function, and supporting the growth and development of cells and tissues. Good sources of vitamin A include carrots, sweet potatoes, spinach, and liver.

Vitamin D: Known as the "sunshine vitamin," vitamin D is synthesized in our skin when exposed to sunlight. It helps regulate calcium and phosphorus absorption, promoting healthy bones and teeth. Vitamin D can also be obtained from fatty fish, fortified dairy products, and egg yolks.

Vitamin E: As a powerful antioxidant, vitamin E protects our cells from damage caused by free radicals. It also plays a role in immune function and helps maintain healthy skin. Good sources of vitamin E include nuts, seeds, vegetable oils, and leafy green vegetables.

Vitamin K: This vitamin is essential for blood clotting and bone health. It helps activate proteins that are involved in the clotting process and supports the deposition of calcium in bones. Leafy green vegetables, broccoli, and soybean oil are good sources of vitamin K.

Water-Soluble Vitamins

B Vitamins: The B vitamins include thiamin (B1), riboflavin (B2), niacin (B3), pantothenic acid (B5), pyridoxine (B6), biotin (B7), folate (B9), and cobalamin (B12). These vitamins play crucial roles in energy metabolism, nerve function, red blood cell production, and DNA synthesis. Good sources of B vitamins include whole grains, legumes, meat, fish, eggs, and leafy green vegetables.

Vitamin C: Also known as ascorbic acid, vitamin C is a powerful antioxidant that supports immune function, collagen synthesis, and iron absorption. Citrus fruits, strawberries, bell peppers, and broccoli are excellent sources of vitamin C.

Minerals

Minerals are inorganic substances that are essential for various physiological processes in our bodies. They can be divided into two categories: macrominerals and trace minerals.

Macrominerals

Calcium: Calcium is crucial for the development and maintenance of strong bones and teeth. It also plays a role in muscle function, nerve transmission, and blood clotting. Dairy products, leafy green vegetables, and fortified foods are good sources of calcium.

Magnesium: This mineral is involved in more than 300 biochemical reactions in our bodies. It helps maintain normal muscle and nerve function, supports a healthy immune system, and regulates blood pressure. Nuts, seeds, whole grains, and leafy green vegetables are rich sources of magnesium.

Potassium: Potassium is essential for maintaining proper fluid balance, nerve function, and muscle contractions. It also helps lower blood pressure and reduce the risk of kidney stones. Bananas, potatoes, avocados, and spinach are good sources of potassium.

Sodium: While sodium is necessary for maintaining proper fluid balance and nerve function, excessive sodium intake can contribute to high blood pressure. It is important to consume sodium in moderation and choose low-sodium options when possible. Processed foods, canned soups, and fast food often contain high levels of sodium.

Trace Minerals

Iron: Iron is essential for the production of hemoglobin, a protein in red blood cells that carries oxygen throughout the body. It also plays a role in energy production and immune function. Good sources of iron include lean meats, seafood, legumes, and fortified cereals.

Zinc: Zinc is involved in numerous enzymatic reactions and plays a crucial role in immune function, wound healing, and DNA synthesis. It can be found in meat, shellfish, legumes, and whole grains.

Iodine: Iodine is necessary for the production of thyroid hormones, which regulate metabolism and growth. Seafood, iodized salt, and dairy products are good sources of iodine.

Selenium: This mineral acts as an antioxidant and is important for thyroid function and DNA synthesis. Brazil nuts, seafood, and whole grains are good sources of selenium.

Copper: Copper is involved in the production of red blood cells, collagen synthesis, and iron absorption. It can be found in organ meats, shellfish, nuts, and seeds.

Manganese: Manganese is necessary for the metabolism of carbohydrates, proteins, and cholesterol. It also acts as an antioxidant. Whole grains, nuts, and leafy green vegetables are good sources of manganese.

Chromium: Chromium plays a role in insulin function and glucose metabolism. It can be found in broccoli, whole grains, and lean meats.

Incorporating a variety of foods rich in vitamins and minerals is essential for meeting our micronutrient needs. A balanced diet that includes fruits, vegetables, whole grains, lean proteins, and dairy products can help ensure an adequate intake of micronutrients. However, it is important to note that individual nutrient needs may vary based on factors such as age, sex, and overall health. Consulting with a healthcare professional or registered dietitian can provide personalized guidance on meeting micronutrient needs through diet and, if necessary, supplementation.

Water

Water is an essential component of a balanced diet and plays a crucial role in maintaining overall health and well-being. It is often referred to as the "elixir of life" because of its numerous benefits and the vital role it plays in various bodily functions. In this section, we will explore the importance of water, how much water you should drink, staying hydrated throughout the day, and hydration tips for exercise and physical activity.

The Role of Water in the Body

Water is the most abundant substance in the human body, making up about 60% of our total body weight. It is involved in almost every physiological process and is essential for the proper functioning of our organs, tissues, and cells. Here are some of the key roles that water plays in our body:

Hydration: Water is the primary component of bodily fluids, including blood, lymph, and digestive juices. It helps transport nutrients, oxygen, and waste products throughout the body.

Temperature regulation: Water helps regulate body temperature through processes like sweating and evaporation. It acts as a coolant, preventing overheating during physical activity or exposure to hot environments.

Digestion and nutrient absorption: Water is necessary for the proper digestion and absorption of nutrients. It helps break down food, aids in the absorption of vitamins and minerals, and facilitates the movement of waste through the digestive system.

Joint lubrication: Water acts as a lubricant for joints, reducing friction and preventing joint pain and stiffness.

Cellular function: Water is involved in various cellular processes, including nutrient uptake, waste removal, and the maintenance of cell structure and function.

Kidney function: Water plays a vital role in kidney function by helping to flush out waste products and toxins from the body through urine.

How Much Water Should You Drink?

The amount of water you need to drink can vary depending on several factors, including your age, sex, activity level, and overall health. While there is no one-size-fits-all answer, a general guideline is to aim for about 8 cups (64 ounces) of water per day. However, individual needs may vary, and it's important to listen to your body's signals of thirst and adjust your intake accordingly.

Here are some factors to consider when determining your water intake:

Activity level: If you engage in physical activity or exercise regularly, you will need to drink more water to compensate for the fluid loss through sweat. It is recommended to drink an additional 1-2 cups of water for every hour of moderate to intense physical activity.

Climate and environment: Hot and humid climates can increase your water needs as you may sweat more. Similarly, high altitudes can also increase water loss through respiration and may require increased hydration.

Health conditions: Certain health conditions, such as kidney stones or urinary tract infections, may require increased water intake as part of the treatment plan. Consult with your healthcare provider for personalized recommendations.

Pregnancy and breastfeeding: Pregnant and breastfeeding women have increased fluid needs to support the growth and development of the baby and to produce breast milk. It is important for them to stay adequately hydrated.

Remember that water intake can come from a variety of sources, including beverages and foods with high water content, such as fruits and vegetables. It's not just about drinking plain water but also incorporating hydrating foods and beverages into your diet.

Staying Hydrated Throughout the Day

Maintaining hydration throughout the day is essential for optimal health and well-being. Here are some tips to help you stay hydrated:

Drink water regularly: Make it a habit to drink water throughout the day, even when you're not feeling thirsty. Carry a reusable water bottle with you to ensure easy access to water wherever you go.

Set reminders: If you often forget to drink water, set reminders on your phone or use apps that can help you track your water intake and send reminders at regular intervals.

Hydrate before, during, and after exercise: Drink water before, during, and after physical activity to replenish fluids lost through sweat and prevent dehydration.

Include hydrating foods: Incorporate foods with high water content, such as watermelon, cucumbers, oranges, and soups, into your meals and snacks.

Limit caffeine and alcohol: Caffeine and alcohol can have a diuretic effect, increasing fluid loss. If you consume these beverages, make sure to balance them with an adequate intake of water.

Pay attention to urine color: Monitor the color of your urine as an indicator of hydration. Pale yellow or clear urine generally indicates adequate hydration, while dark yellow urine may be a sign of dehydration.

Hydration Tips for Exercise and Physical Activity

Proper hydration is especially important during exercise and physical activity to maintain performance, prevent fatigue, and avoid dehydration. Here are some tips to stay hydrated during exercise:

Pre-hydrate: Drink water before starting your workout to ensure you are adequately hydrated.

Drink during exercise: Sip water throughout your workout, especially during intense or prolonged exercise sessions. Aim to drink about 1 cup (8 ounces) of water every 15-20 minutes.

Consider electrolyte replacement: If you engage in prolonged or intense exercise, consider consuming sports drinks or electrolyte-rich beverages to replenish electrolytes lost through sweat.

Rehydrate post-workout: Drink water after your workout to replace any fluids lost during exercise.

Remember that individual hydration needs can vary based on factors such as exercise intensity, duration, and sweat rate. It's important to listen to your body and adjust your fluid intake accordingly.

In conclusion, water is a vital component of a balanced diet and plays a crucial role in maintaining overall health and well-being. It is essential for hydration, temperature regulation, digestion, joint lubrication, cellular function, and kidney function. The amount of water you need to drink can vary based on factors such as age, sex, activity level, and health conditions. Staying hydrated throughout the day and during exercise is important for optimal health and performance. Incorporate these tips into your daily routine to ensure you meet your body's water needs and stay properly hydrated.

Understanding Nutrient Labels

Nutrient labels are an essential tool for understanding the nutritional content of the food we consume. They provide valuable information about the macronutrients, micronutrients, and other components present in a particular food product. By reading and understanding nutrient labels, we can make informed choices about the foods we eat and ensure that we are meeting our nutritional needs.

Importance of Nutrient Labels

Nutrient labels play a crucial role in helping us maintain a balanced diet. They provide detailed information about the amount of calories, fats, carbohydrates, proteins, vitamins, minerals, and other nutrients present in a serving of food. This information allows us to assess the nutritional value of a product and make comparisons between different options.

Understanding nutrient labels is particularly important for individuals with specific dietary requirements or health conditions. For example, someone with diabetes may need to monitor their carbohydrate intake, while someone with high blood pressure may need to limit their sodium consumption. Nutrient labels can help these individuals make informed choices and manage their conditions effectively.

Components of Nutrient Labels

To effectively understand nutrient labels, it is essential to familiarize ourselves with the different components they contain. Here are the key elements typically found on nutrient labels:

Serving Size: This indicates the recommended portion size for the food product. It is important to note that the nutritional information provided on the label is based on this serving size.

Calories: This section provides information about the number of calories present in one serving of the food. Calories are a measure of the energy content of the food.

Macronutrients: Nutrient labels also provide information about the macronutrients present in the food, including fats, carbohydrates, and proteins. These are typically listed in grams and as a percentage of the recommended daily intake.

Micronutrients: The label may also include information about the presence of vitamins, minerals, and other micronutrients. These are usually listed as a percentage of the recommended daily intake.

Ingredients: This section lists all the ingredients present in the food product, starting with the most abundant ingredient. It is important to review this section, especially if you have any allergies or dietary restrictions.

Allergen Information: Nutrient labels often highlight the presence of common allergens such as peanuts, tree nuts, soy, wheat, dairy, and shellfish. This information is crucial for individuals with food allergies or intolerances.

Additional Information: Some nutrient labels may provide additional information, such as dietary fiber content, sugar content, cholesterol levels, and sodium levels. These details can be helpful for individuals who need to monitor specific nutrients.

Interpreting Nutrient Labels

Interpreting nutrient labels can be overwhelming at first, but with practice, it becomes easier to make sense of the information provided. Here are some tips to help you understand and interpret nutrient labels effectively:

Compare Similar Products: When shopping for food, compare the nutrient labels of different brands or varieties of the same product. This will allow you to choose the option that best aligns with your nutritional goals.

Pay Attention to Serving Sizes: Remember that the nutritional information on the label is based on the serving size mentioned. If you consume more or less than the recommended serving size, you will need to adjust the nutrient values accordingly.

Check the Percent Daily Value (%DV): The %DV indicates how much of a particular nutrient one serving of the food contributes to your daily recommended intake. Aim for foods that provide a higher %DV of essential nutrients like vitamins and minerals.

Consider Your Individual Needs: Keep in mind that nutrient needs vary depending on factors such as age, sex, activity level, and overall health. Adjust your food choices based on your specific requirements.

Look for Hidden Ingredients: Nutrient labels can help you identify hidden ingredients such as added sugars, unhealthy fats, and artificial additives. Be mindful of these components and choose products with minimal or no added sugars and unhealthy fats.

Use Nutrient Labels for Meal Planning: Nutrient labels can be a valuable tool for meal planning. By understanding the nutritional content of different foods, you can create well-balanced meals that meet your specific dietary needs.

Seek Professional Guidance: If you have specific dietary concerns or health conditions, it is always advisable to consult a registered dietitian or healthcare professional. They can provide personalized guidance and help you interpret nutrient labels in the context of your unique needs.

By understanding and utilizing nutrient labels effectively, we can make informed choices about the foods we consume and ensure that our diet is balanced and nutritionally adequate. Incorporating this knowledge into our daily lives empowers us to take control of our health and well-being.

CALORIE NEEDS OF DIFFERENT INDIVIDUALS

Factors Affecting Calorie Needs

Calories are a measure of the energy provided by food and beverages. The number of calories a person needs each day can vary based on several factors. Understanding these factors is crucial for determining an individual's calorie needs and maintaining a balanced diet.

Metabolic Rate

One of the primary factors affecting calorie needs is an individual's metabolic rate. Metabolism refers to the chemical processes that occur within the body to maintain life. The basal metabolic rate (BMR) is the number of calories the body needs to perform basic functions at rest, such as breathing, circulating blood, and maintaining body temperature.

Several factors influence an individual's metabolic rate, including age, gender, body composition, and genetics. Generally, younger individuals tend to have a higher metabolic rate compared to older individuals. Men typically have a higher BMR than women due to differences in muscle mass and hormonal factors. Additionally, individuals with more muscle mass tend to have a higher metabolic rate than those with higher body fat percentages.

Physical Activity Level

Another crucial factor affecting calorie needs is the level of physical activity. Physical activity includes any movement of the body that requires energy expenditure, such as exercise, household chores, or even walking to work. The more physically active a person is, the more calories they will burn.

Different types and intensities of physical activity have varying calorie-burning effects. For example, high-intensity exercises like running or weightlifting burn more calories per minute compared to low-intensity activities like walking or stretching. Additionally, the duration and frequency of physical activity also play a role in determining calorie needs.

Body Composition

Body composition refers to the proportion of fat, muscle, bone, and other tissues in the body. It is an essential factor in determining calorie needs. Muscle tissue is more metabolically active than fat tissue, meaning it burns more calories at rest. Therefore, individuals with a higher percentage of muscle mass generally have a higher metabolic rate and require more calories to maintain their weight.

On the other hand, individuals with a higher percentage of body fat may have a lower metabolic rate and require fewer calories. It is important to note that body composition can vary significantly among individuals, even if they have the same weight and height. Therefore, it is crucial to consider body composition when determining calorie needs.

Age and Growth

Calorie needs also vary based on age and growth. Children and adolescents have higher calorie needs compared to adults due to their rapid growth and development. During growth spurts, their bodies require additional energy to support the development of bones, muscles, and organs. It is essential for children and adolescents to consume a balanced diet to meet their increased calorie needs and ensure proper growth and development.

As individuals age, their calorie needs may decrease due to a decrease in muscle mass and a decrease in physical activity levels. However, it is important to note that older adults still require adequate nutrition to support their overall health and prevent age-related conditions.

Health Conditions

Certain health conditions can affect an individual's calorie needs. For example, individuals with a higher metabolic rate due to conditions like hyperthyroidism may require more calories to maintain their weight. On the other hand, individuals with conditions that affect digestion or nutrient absorption, such as celiac disease or Crohn's disease, may have increased nutrient needs but may struggle to consume enough calories.

Additionally, individuals recovering from surgery or illness may have increased calorie needs to support the healing process. It is important for individuals with specific health conditions to work with healthcare professionals or registered dietitians to determine their individual calorie needs and ensure they are meeting their nutritional requirements.

Environmental Factors

Environmental factors can also influence calorie needs. For example, individuals living in colder climates may require more calories to maintain body temperature due to increased energy expenditure. Similarly, individuals engaged in physically demanding occupations, such as construction workers or athletes, may have higher calorie needs to fuel their activities.

Conclusion

Understanding the factors that affect calorie needs is essential for maintaining a balanced diet and overall health. Factors such as metabolic rate, physical activity level, body composition, age, growth, health conditions, and environmental factors all play a role in determining an individual's calorie needs. By considering these factors, individuals can make informed decisions about their dietary choices and ensure they are consuming the appropriate amount of calories to support their unique needs.

Calculating Basal Metabolic Rate (BMR)

Basal Metabolic Rate (BMR) is the number of calories your body needs to perform basic functions while at rest. These functions include breathing, circulating blood, regulating body temperature, and maintaining organ function. Calculating your BMR is an essential step in determining your daily calorie needs and creating a balanced diet plan that supports your health goals.

There are several formulas available to estimate BMR, but one of the most commonly used is the Harris-Benedict equation. This equation takes into account your age, gender, weight, and height to calculate your BMR. Here is the formula for men and women:

For men: BMR = 88.362 + (13.397 × weight in kg) + (4.799 × height in cm) - (5.677 × age in years)

For women: BMR = 447.593 + (9.247 × weight in kg) + (3.098 × height in cm) - (4.330 × age in years)

Let's break down the formula and understand each component:

Weight: Your weight is an important factor in determining your BMR. The more you weigh, the more calories your body needs to maintain its basic functions.

Height: Your height also plays a role in calculating your BMR. Taller individuals generally have a higher BMR compared to shorter individuals.

Age: As you age, your BMR tends to decrease. This is because as you get older, your body tends to lose muscle mass and gain fat, which slows down your metabolism.

Gender: Men generally have a higher BMR compared to women. This is because men tend to have more muscle mass, which requires more calories to maintain.

Now, let's take an example to understand how to calculate BMR:

Sarah is a 30-year-old woman who weighs 65 kilograms and is 165 centimeters tall. To calculate her BMR, we will use the formula for women:

BMR = 447.593 + (9.247 × 65) + (3.098 × 165) - (4.330 × 30)

BMR = 447.593 + 601.255 + 509.67 - 129.9

BMR = 1428.618

Sarah's BMR is approximately 1428.618 calories per day. This means that if Sarah were to lie in bed all day without any physical activity, her body would require around 1428.618 calories to perform basic functions.

It's important to note that BMR is just an estimate and individual variations can occur. Factors such as muscle mass, body composition, and overall health can influence your BMR. Additionally, BMR does not take into account your activity level, which is crucial in determining your total daily calorie needs.

To determine your total daily calorie needs, you need to multiply your BMR by an activity factor that represents your level of physical activity. The activity factors are as follows:

Sedentary (little to no exercise): BMR × 1.2

Lightly active (light exercise/sports 1-3 days a week): BMR × 1.375

Moderately active (moderate exercise/sports 3-5 days a week): BMR × 1.55

Very active (hard exercise/sports 6-7 days a week): BMR × 1.725

Extra active (very hard exercise/sports and a physical job): BMR × 1.9

For example, if Sarah is moderately active, we would multiply her BMR by 1.55 to determine her total daily calorie needs.

Total daily calorie needs = BMR × Activity Factor

Total daily calorie needs = 1428.618 × 1.55

Total daily calorie needs = 2213.9

Therefore, Sarah's total daily calorie needs would be approximately 2213.9 calories per day to maintain her current weight and activity level.

Calculating your BMR and total daily calorie needs is an important step in creating a balanced diet plan that supports your health goals. It provides a baseline for determining the appropriate calorie intake and helps you make informed decisions about the types and quantities of food you consume. Remember, these calculations are just estimates, and it's always a good idea to consult with a healthcare professional or registered dietitian for personalized guidance.

Determining Daily Calorie Intake

Determining your daily calorie intake is an essential step in achieving a balanced diet. The number of calories you need each day depends on various factors, including your age, gender, weight, height, activity level, and overall health goals. By understanding how to calculate your daily calorie needs, you can ensure that you are providing your body with the right amount of energy to function optimally.

Factors Affecting Calorie Needs

Several factors influence your daily calorie needs. These factors include:

Basal Metabolic Rate (BMR): Your BMR is the number of calories your body needs to perform basic functions such as breathing, circulating blood, and maintaining body temperature while at rest. It accounts for the largest portion of your daily calorie expenditure, typically around 60-75%.

Physical Activity Level: The amount of physical activity you engage in throughout the day affects your calorie needs. Those who lead a sedentary lifestyle require fewer calories compared to individuals who are physically active or engage in regular exercise.

Age and Gender: Age and gender play a role in determining your calorie needs. Generally, men tend to have higher calorie requirements than women due to differences in body composition and muscle mass. Additionally, calorie needs may decrease with age as metabolism naturally slows down.

Body Composition: Your body composition, including the amount of muscle mass and fat, affects your calorie needs. Muscle tissue is more metabolically active than fat tissue, meaning that individuals with higher muscle mass generally have higher calorie requirements.

Health Conditions: Certain health conditions, such as thyroid disorders or metabolic disorders, can affect your metabolism and, consequently, your calorie needs. It is important to consult with a healthcare professional if you have any underlying health conditions that may impact your calorie intake.

Calculating Basal Metabolic Rate (BMR)

To determine your BMR, you can use various formulas, such as the Harris-Benedict equation or the

Mifflin-St Jeor equation. These formulas take into account your age, gender, weight, and height to estimate your BMR. However, keep in mind that these formulas provide an estimate, and individual variations may exist.

For example, the Harris-Benedict equation for calculating BMR is as follows:

For men: BMR = 88.362 + (13.397 × weight in kg) + (4.799 × height in cm) - (5.677 × age in years)

For women: BMR = 447.593 + (9.247 × weight in kg) + (3.098 × height in cm) - (4.330 × age in years)

Once you have calculated your BMR, you can use it as a starting point to determine your daily calorie needs.

Determining Daily Calorie Intake

To determine your daily calorie intake, you need to consider your BMR and activity level. The BMR provides an estimate of the calories needed for basic bodily functions, while the activity level accounts for additional calories burned through physical activity.

To estimate your daily calorie needs, you can multiply your BMR by an activity factor:

Sedentary (little to no exercise): BMR × 1.2

Lightly active (light exercise/sports 1-3 days per week): BMR × 1.375

Moderately active (moderate exercise/sports 3-5 days per week): BMR × 1.55

Very active (hard exercise/sports 6-7 days per week): BMR × 1.725

Extra active (very hard exercise/sports and a physical job): BMR × 1.9

For example, if your BMR is 1500 calories and you engage in moderate exercise 3-5 days per week, your estimated daily calorie intake would be 1500 × 1.55 = 2325 calories.

It is important to note that these calculations provide a general estimate and may need to be adjusted based on individual factors and goals. If you are looking to lose weight, you may need to create a calorie deficit by consuming fewer calories than your estimated daily intake. Conversely, if you are looking to gain weight or build muscle, you may need to consume more calories.

Adjusting Calorie Intake for Weight Management

If your goal is weight management, you can adjust your calorie intake accordingly. To lose weight, you need to create a calorie deficit by consuming fewer calories than your body needs. A safe and sustainable rate of weight loss is generally around 0.5-1 pound per week, which requires a calorie deficit of approximately 500-1000 calories per day.

On the other hand, if your goal is to gain weight or build muscle, you need to create a calorie surplus by consuming more calories than your body needs. This surplus provides the extra energy required for muscle growth and repair. It is important to focus on consuming nutrient-dense foods to support overall health and avoid excessive weight gain from unhealthy sources.

Remember that weight management is a gradual process, and it is essential to prioritize overall health and well-being rather than solely focusing on the number on the scale. Consulting with a registered dietitian or healthcare professional can provide personalized guidance and support in achieving your weight management goals while maintaining a balanced diet.

Determining your daily calorie intake is a crucial step in achieving a balanced diet. By understanding the factors that influence your calorie needs and using appropriate calculations, you can ensure that you are providing your body with the right amount of energy to support optimal health and well-being.

Adjusting Calorie Intake for Weight Management

When it comes to weight management, adjusting your calorie intake is a crucial aspect of achieving your goals. Whether you want to lose weight, gain weight, or maintain your current weight, understanding how to adjust your calorie intake is essential. In this section, we will explore the different strategies and considerations for adjusting your calorie intake for weight management.

Understanding Calorie Balance

Before we delve into the specifics of adjusting calorie intake, it's important to understand the concept of calorie balance. Calorie balance refers to the relationship between the calories you consume through food and beverages and the calories you burn through physical activity and bodily functions. When you consume more calories than you burn, you are in a state of positive calorie balance, which can lead to weight gain. Conversely, when you burn more calories than you consume, you are in a state of negative calorie balance, which can result in weight loss.

Determining Your Calorie Needs

To adjust your calorie intake for weight management, you first need to determine your daily calorie needs. Several factors influence your calorie needs, including age, gender, weight, height, activity level, and overall health. One commonly used method to estimate calorie needs is the Harris-Benedict equation, which calculates your Basal Metabolic Rate (BMR) – the number of calories your body needs to perform basic functions at rest. Once you have your BMR, you can multiply it by an activity factor to estimate your total daily calorie needs.

For example, let's consider a 35-year-old woman who weighs 150 pounds, is 5'6" tall, and exercises moderately three to four times a week. Using the Harris-Benedict equation, her estimated BMR would be approximately 1,400 calories. If we multiply this by an activity factor of 1.55 (moderate activity level), her total daily calorie needs would be around 2,170 calories.

Adjusting Calorie Intake for Weight Loss

If your goal is to lose weight, you need to create a calorie deficit by consuming fewer calories than you burn. It's generally recommended to aim for a gradual and sustainable weight loss of 1-2 pounds per week. To achieve this, you can start by reducing your daily calorie intake by 500-1000 calories. This deficit can be achieved through a combination of dietary changes and increased physical activity.

For example, if our 35-year-old woman from the previous example wants to lose weight, she could aim for a daily calorie intake of around 1,670-1,670 calories. This deficit of 500-1000 calories per day would result in a weekly weight loss of 1-2 pounds.

Adjusting Calorie Intake for Weight Gain

On the other hand, if your goal is to gain weight, you need to create a calorie surplus by consuming more calories than you burn. This surplus should come from nutrient-dense foods to ensure you are gaining healthy weight. It's important to focus on increasing your calorie intake gradually and incorporating strength training exercises to promote muscle growth.

For example, let's consider a 25-year-old man who wants to gain weight. If his estimated daily calorie needs are 2,500 calories, he could aim to consume an additional 300-500 calories per day to create a calorie surplus. This surplus, combined with a strength training program, can help him gain weight in the form of muscle mass.

Monitoring and Adjusting

Once you have adjusted your calorie intake for weight management, it's crucial to monitor your progress and make adjustments as needed. Keep track of your food intake and physical activity to ensure you are staying on track with your goals. If you are not seeing the desired results, you may need to further adjust your calorie intake or reassess your activity level.

It's important to note that individual responses to calorie adjustments may vary. Factors such as genetics, metabolism, and overall health can influence how your body responds to changes in calorie intake. It's always a good idea to consult with a healthcare professional or registered dietitian before making significant changes to your calorie intake or embarking on a weight management journey.

In conclusion, adjusting your calorie intake is a fundamental aspect of weight management. Whether your goal is to lose weight, gain weight, or maintain your current weight, understanding your calorie needs and creating an appropriate calorie balance is key. By making gradual and sustainable adjustments to your calorie intake, combined with a balanced diet and regular physical activity, you can achieve your weight management goals and maintain a healthy lifestyle.

PORTION CONTROL

Understanding Portion Sizes

Portion control is an essential aspect of maintaining a balanced diet. It involves understanding and managing the amount of food you consume in each meal or snack. By practicing portion control, you can ensure that you are providing your body with the right amount of nutrients while avoiding overeating and unnecessary weight gain.

Understanding portion sizes is crucial because it helps you gauge how much food you should be consuming to meet your nutritional needs. Many people struggle with portion control because they are not aware of what constitutes a proper serving size. It is common for individuals to underestimate the amount of food they consume, leading to excessive calorie intake and potential health issues.

To better understand portion sizes, it is helpful to familiarize yourself with some common measurements and visual cues. Here are a few examples:

Hand measurements: Your hand can serve as a useful tool for estimating portion sizes. For instance, a serving of protein (such as chicken or fish) should be about the size of your palm. A serving of carbohydrates (like rice or pasta) should be approximately the size of your clenched fist. And a serving of fats (such as nuts or oils) should be about the size of your thumb.

Visual cues: Visual cues can also assist you in determining appropriate portion sizes. For example, a serving of vegetables should be roughly the size of a baseball or your closed fist. A serving of fruit is typically equivalent to a tennis ball. When it comes to grains, such as bread or cereal, one serving is approximately the size of a hockey puck.

Measuring tools: Using measuring cups, spoons, and a kitchen scale can provide more accurate measurements for portion control. Measuring cups can help you determine the appropriate amount of grains, liquids, and other ingredients. Measuring spoons are useful for portioning out condiments, oils, and spices. A kitchen scale can be particularly helpful for weighing proteins, such as meat or fish, to ensure you are consuming the recommended serving size.

It is important to note that portion sizes may vary depending on your individual needs and goals. Factors such as age, gender, activity level, and overall health can influence the amount of food you should consume. Consulting with a registered dietitian or healthcare professional can provide personalized guidance on portion control based on your specific requirements.

Practicing portion control does not mean you have to deprive yourself or restrict your food intake. It is about finding a balance and making conscious choices about the quantity of food you consume. Here are some tips to help you maintain portion control:

Read food labels: Pay attention to serving sizes listed on food labels. This information can help you understand how much of a particular food constitutes one serving. Be mindful of the number of servings you consume to avoid exceeding your intended portion size.

Use smaller plates and bowls: Opt for smaller plates and bowls when serving your meals. Research suggests that using smaller dishware can trick your brain into perceiving larger portions, leading to a feeling of satisfaction with less food.

Divide your plate: Visualize your plate divided into sections. Fill half of your plate with vegetables, one-quarter with lean protein, and one-quarter with whole grains or starchy vegetables. This method can help you create balanced meals and control portion sizes.

Practice mindful eating: Slow down and pay attention to your body's hunger and fullness cues. Eating slowly and savoring each bite can help you feel more satisfied with smaller portions. Avoid distractions, such as television or electronic devices, while eating to focus on your meal.

Pre-portion snacks: Instead of eating directly from a large bag or container, pre-portion snacks into smaller containers or bags. This strategy can prevent mindless eating and help you stick to appropriate portion sizes.

Be aware of restaurant portions: Restaurant meals often come in larger portions than what is necessary for one sitting. Consider sharing a meal with a friend or asking for a takeout container to save the excess for another meal. You can also choose appetizers or half-size portions when available.

By understanding portion sizes and implementing portion control strategies, you can maintain a balanced diet and support your overall health and well-being. Remember, it is not just about what you eat but also how much you eat that contributes to a healthy lifestyle.

Tips for Portion Control

Portion control plays a crucial role in maintaining a balanced diet. It involves managing the amount of food you consume to ensure that you are eating the right portions for your body's needs. By practicing portion control, you can prevent overeating, maintain a healthy weight, and improve your overall well-being. Here are some practical tips to help you master portion control:

Use smaller plates and bowls: The size of your dinnerware can influence how much you eat. By using smaller plates and bowls, you can trick your mind into thinking that you are consuming a larger portion. This visual illusion can help you feel satisfied with less food.

Measure your food: It's easy to underestimate portion sizes, especially when it comes to calorie-dense foods. To avoid overeating, use measuring cups, spoons, or a food scale to accurately measure your food. This practice will give you a better understanding of appropriate portion sizes.

Be mindful of serving sizes: Familiarize yourself with standard serving sizes for different food groups. For example, a serving of cooked pasta is typically half a cup, while a serving of meat is about the size of a deck of cards. Understanding these guidelines can help you gauge appropriate portion sizes when serving yourself.

Fill half your plate with vegetables: Vegetables are low in calories and high in nutrients, making them an excellent choice for portion control. Aim to fill half of your plate with a variety of colorful vegetables. This not only helps control portion sizes but also ensures you are getting a good balance of vitamins and minerals.

Practice the "handy" portion guide: Your hand can serve as a handy tool for estimating portion sizes. For example, a serving of protein (such as chicken or fish) should be about the size of your palm. A cupped hand can represent a serving of grains or starchy vegetables, while a thumb can be used to measure fats and oils.

Slow down and savor your food: Eating mindfully and savoring each bite can help you recognize when you are full. Take the time to chew your food thoroughly and pay attention to your body's hunger and fullness cues. This practice can prevent overeating and promote better digestion.

Pre-portion your snacks: Snacking can easily lead to mindless eating and overconsumption. To avoid this, pre-portion your snacks into individual servings. This way, you can grab a single portion without the temptation to eat more than you intended.

Limit liquid calories: Beverages such as soda, fruit juices, and alcoholic drinks can contribute a significant amount of calories to your diet. Be mindful of liquid calories and opt for healthier alternatives like water, herbal tea, or infused water with fruits and herbs.

Be aware of hidden calories: Some foods may appear healthy but can be high in calories. Pay attention to dressings, sauces, and condiments, as they can add extra calories to your meals. Consider using smaller amounts or opting for lower-calorie alternatives.

Plan and prepare your meals: Planning and preparing your meals in advance can help you control portion sizes. By cooking at home, you have more control over the ingredients and portion sizes. Additionally, packing your lunch and snacks for work or outings can prevent impulsive and oversized food choices.

Listen to your body's hunger and fullness cues: It's essential to tune in to your body's signals of hunger and fullness. Eat when you are hungry and stop when you are satisfied, not overly full. This mindful approach to eating can help you maintain a healthy weight and prevent overeating.

Seek support and accountability: Changing your eating habits can be challenging, but having support and accountability can make a significant difference. Consider joining a support group, working with a registered dietitian, or involving a friend or family member in your journey towards portion control.

Remember, portion control is not about depriving yourself of food but rather about finding a balance that works for your body and health goals. By implementing these tips and practicing mindful eating, you can develop a healthier relationship with food and maintain a balanced diet.

Portion Control for Dining Out

Dining out can be a challenge when it comes to maintaining portion control and making healthy choices. Restaurants often serve large portions, which can lead to overeating and consuming more calories than necessary. However, with a few strategies and mindful choices, you can still enjoy dining out while staying on track with your balanced diet goals.

Understanding Portion Sizes

Before we delve into the tips for portion control while dining out, it's important to understand what appropriate portion sizes look like. Portion sizes can vary depending on the type of food and the individual's calorie needs. Here are some general guidelines to keep in mind:

Protein: A serving of protein, such as chicken, fish, or tofu, should be about the size of a deck of cards or the palm of your hand.

Grains: A serving of grains, such as rice or pasta, should be about the size of your fist or a tennis ball.

Vegetables: Aim to fill half of your plate with non-starchy vegetables, such as broccoli, spinach, or peppers.

Fruits: A serving of fruit is typically the size of a tennis ball or a small piece of fruit, like an apple or orange.

Fats: Healthy fats, such as avocado or nuts, should be consumed in moderation. A serving of fats is about the size of a thumb.

Tips for Portion Control

Now that you have a better understanding of portion sizes, let's explore some practical tips for portion control while dining out:

Choose smaller portions: Look for options on the menu that offer smaller portion sizes or half portions. Many restaurants now offer healthier alternatives or "light" menu options that are designed with portion control in mind.

Share your meal: Consider splitting an entrée with a dining partner or asking for a to-go box at the beginning of the meal and portioning out half of your meal to take home. This way, you can enjoy your favorite dishes without overeating.

Be mindful of appetizers and sides: Appetizers and side dishes can add extra calories and increase portion sizes. Opt for healthier options like a salad or steamed vegetables instead of fried or creamy appetizers.

Ask for dressings and sauces on the side: Many dressings and sauces are high in calories and can quickly add up. Request them on the side, and use them sparingly to control the amount you consume.

Fill up on vegetables: When ordering, prioritize dishes that are rich in vegetables. They are low in calories and high in nutrients, helping you feel satisfied without overindulging in higher-calorie options.

Avoid all-you-can-eat buffets: Buffets can be tempting, but they often encourage overeating due to the wide variety and unlimited portions. If you do find yourself at a buffet, focus on filling your plate with vegetables, lean proteins, and smaller portions of higher-calorie foods.

Be cautious with beverages: Many beverages, such as sodas, juices, and alcoholic drinks, can be high in calories. Opt for water, unsweetened tea, or sparkling water with a splash of citrus instead.

Practice mindful eating: Slow down and savor each bite. Pay attention to your body's hunger and fullness cues. Stop eating when you feel satisfied, even if there is food left on your plate.

Portion Control Tools and Techniques

In addition to the tips mentioned above, there are several tools and techniques that can assist you in practicing portion control while dining out:

Use smaller plates: If you have the option, choose a smaller plate or bowl. Research has shown that people tend to eat less when they use smaller plates, as it creates the illusion of a fuller plate.

Measure and estimate portions: If you have a good sense of portion sizes, you can estimate them visually. However, if you're unsure, consider carrying a small measuring cup or using your hand as a guide. For example, a cupped hand can approximate a serving of nuts or a tablespoon of nut butter.

Take note of visual cues: Pay attention to the visual cues provided by the restaurant. Some establishments may offer portion-controlled meals or indicate the appropriate serving size on the menu. Look for keywords like "light," "healthy," or "portion-controlled" when making your selection.

Practice self-control: It's essential to develop self-control and resist the temptation to indulge in larger portions or unhealthy choices. Remind yourself of your goals and the importance of maintaining a balanced diet.

By implementing these portion control strategies and techniques, you can enjoy dining out while still adhering to your balanced diet. Remember, it's all about making mindful choices, being aware of portion sizes, and listening to your body's hunger and fullness cues. With practice, portion control will become second nature, allowing you to maintain a healthy and balanced lifestyle even when dining out.

Portion Control Tools and Techniques

Portion control is an essential aspect of maintaining a balanced diet. It involves managing the amount of food you consume to ensure that you are eating appropriate portions for your body's needs. While it may seem challenging at first, there are various tools and techniques available to help you achieve portion control effectively. In this section, we will explore some of these tools and techniques that can assist you in managing your portion sizes and making healthier choices.

Portion Control Plates

One popular tool for portion control is the portion control plate. These plates are designed with sections that indicate the appropriate proportions of different food groups. By using a portion control plate, you can visually understand how much of each food group you should be consuming in a single meal. For example, a typical portion control plate may have sections for vegetables, proteins, carbohydrates, and fats. By filling each section with the recommended amount of food, you can ensure that you are consuming a well-balanced meal.

Measuring Cups and Spoons

Measuring cups and spoons are simple yet effective tools for portion control. By using these tools, you can accurately measure the amount of food you are consuming. For example, if a recipe calls for one cup of rice, using a measuring cup ensures that you are not unknowingly consuming more than the recommended portion. Measuring spoons are particularly useful for ingredients such as oils, dressings, and spices, where even a small amount can significantly impact the overall calorie and nutrient content of a dish.

Food Scales

Food scales are another valuable tool for portion control, especially when it comes to measuring solid foods. By weighing your food, you can accurately determine the portion size and ensure that you are not overeating. For example, if a serving of chicken is 4 ounces, using a food scale allows you to measure the exact amount you are consuming. Food scales are particularly helpful for individuals who are trying to manage their calorie intake or follow specific dietary guidelines.

Portion Control Containers

Portion control containers are a convenient and portable option for managing portion sizes. These containers are pre-portioned and labeled with the recommended serving sizes for different food groups. By using portion control containers, you can easily pack your meals and snacks for the day, ensuring that you are consuming the right amount of each food group. This method is particularly useful for individuals who are always on the go or struggle with estimating portion sizes.

Visual References

Developing a visual reference for portion sizes can be a helpful technique for portion control. For example, a deck of cards can serve as a reference for a recommended serving size of meat or poultry. A tennis ball can represent a serving of fruit, and a hockey puck can indicate the appropriate portion of carbohydrates. By associating these visual references with specific food groups, you can quickly gauge the appropriate portion sizes without relying on measuring tools.

Mindful Eating

Practicing mindful eating is a technique that can help you control your portion sizes and make healthier food choices. Mindful eating involves paying attention to your body's hunger and fullness cues and eating slowly and consciously. By savoring each bite and being aware of your body's signals, you can better gauge when you are satisfied and avoid overeating. This technique encourages you to focus on the quality of the food you are consuming and promotes a more balanced and mindful approach to eating.

Plate Size and Portion Distortion

The size of your plate can significantly impact your portion sizes. Research has shown that individuals tend to consume more food when using larger plates, as it creates an optical illusion of smaller portions. By using smaller plates and bowls, you can visually trick your mind into perceiving larger portions, even when you are consuming appropriate amounts. Additionally, being mindful of portion distortion, which refers to the gradual increase in portion sizes over time, can help you make conscious choices and avoid overeating.

Restaurant Strategies

When dining out, it can be challenging to control portion sizes, as restaurants often serve larger portions than necessary. However, there are strategies you can employ to manage your portions effectively. One technique is to ask for a to-go box at the beginning of the meal and immediately portion out half of your meal to take home. This way, you can enjoy your meal without feeling obligated to finish the entire portion. Additionally, sharing a meal with a dining partner or ordering appetizers as your main course can help control portion sizes.

Tracking Apps and Journals

Utilizing tracking apps or keeping a food journal can be beneficial for portion control. These tools allow you to record and monitor your food intake, making you more aware of your portion sizes and overall calorie consumption. By tracking your meals, you can identify patterns, make adjustments, and hold yourself accountable for your portion choices. Many tracking apps also provide nutritional information, making it easier to track your macronutrient and micronutrient intake.

Incorporating these portion control tools and techniques into your daily routine can help you develop healthier eating habits and maintain a balanced diet. Remember, portion control is not about depriving yourself but rather about making conscious choices and finding the right balance for your body's needs.

FOOD GROUPS

The Five Food Groups

A balanced diet is not just about eating a variety of foods, but also about ensuring that you consume the right proportions of each food group. The five food groups provide essential nutrients that our bodies need to function properly. By understanding these food groups and incorporating them into our meals, we can achieve a well-rounded and nutritious diet.

The Five Food Groups

Fruits: Fruits are not only delicious but also packed with vitamins, minerals, and fiber. They provide essential nutrients that help support our immune system, promote healthy skin, and aid in digestion. Examples of fruits include apples, oranges, bananas, berries, and melons. It is recommended to consume a variety of fruits to ensure a wide range of nutrients.

Vegetables: Vegetables are a vital part of a balanced diet as they are low in calories and high in nutrients. They provide essential vitamins, minerals, and fiber that support overall health and well-being. Examples of vegetables include leafy greens like spinach and kale, cruciferous vegetables like broccoli and cauliflower, and root vegetables like carrots and potatoes. Aim to include a variety of vegetables in your meals to maximize nutrient intake.

Grains: Grains are a significant source of energy and provide essential nutrients such as carbohydrates, fiber, and B vitamins. Whole grains, such as brown rice, whole wheat bread, and quinoa, are preferred over refined grains as they retain more nutrients and fiber. Incorporating grains into your diet can help maintain energy levels and support proper digestion.

Proteins: Proteins are the building blocks of our bodies and are essential for growth, repair, and maintenance of tissues. They also play a crucial role in the production of enzymes, hormones, and antibodies. Good sources of protein include lean meats, poultry, fish, eggs, dairy products, legumes, and nuts. Including a variety of protein sources in your diet ensures that you receive all the essential amino acids your body needs.

Dairy and Alternatives: Dairy products are excellent sources of calcium, protein, and other essential nutrients. However, if you are lactose intolerant or follow a vegan diet, there are alternatives available. Examples of dairy alternatives include soy milk, almond milk, and tofu. These alternatives are often fortified with calcium and other nutrients to provide similar benefits to dairy products.

Building a Balanced Plate

To create a balanced meal, it is important to include foods from each of the five food groups. One way to visualize this is by using the concept of a balanced plate. Imagine dividing your plate into four sections:

Fill half of your plate with fruits and vegetables. This ensures that you are getting a good amount of vitamins, minerals, and fiber. Aim for a variety of colors to maximize nutrient intake.

Allocate a quarter of your plate for grains. Choose whole grains whenever possible, as they provide more nutrients and fiber compared to refined grains. Examples include whole wheat bread, brown rice, and whole grain pasta.

Reserve the remaining quarter of your plate for proteins. Include lean meats, poultry, fish, legumes, or tofu. These options provide essential amino acids and other nutrients necessary for optimal health.

Alongside your plate, include a serving of dairy or a dairy alternative. This can be a glass of milk, a cup of yogurt, or a serving of cheese. If you prefer dairy alternatives, choose fortified options to ensure you are still getting essential nutrients like calcium.

By following this balanced plate approach, you can ensure that you are consuming a variety of nutrients from each food group, promoting overall health and well-being.

Sample Meal Plans for Different Food Groups

To further illustrate how to incorporate the five food groups into your meals, here are some sample meal plans:

Breakfast: Start your day with a bowl of oatmeal topped with fresh berries (fruits) and a sprinkle of nuts (proteins). Enjoy a glass of milk or a dairy alternative on the side.

Lunch: Prepare a salad with mixed greens (vegetables), grilled chicken (proteins), and a side of quinoa (grains). Add some sliced avocado for healthy fats. Pair it with a piece of fruit for dessert.

Snack: Enjoy a handful of baby carrots (vegetables) with hummus (proteins) for a nutritious and satisfying snack.

Dinner: Grill a salmon fillet (proteins) and serve it with a side of roasted vegetables (vegetables) and a portion of brown rice (grains). Finish the meal with a serving of yogurt or a dairy alternative for dessert.

Remember, these are just examples, and you can mix and match foods from different food groups to create your own balanced meals. The key is to ensure that you are including a variety of nutrients from each food group throughout the day.

Food Group Substitutions and Alternatives

While it is important to include foods from each food group, it is also essential to consider individual dietary preferences, allergies, and intolerances. Here are some food group substitutions and alternatives:

Fruits and Vegetables: If you have specific allergies or intolerances, you can substitute fruits and vegetables with options that suit your needs. For example, if you are allergic to bananas, you can replace them with other fruits like apples or oranges. If you are intolerant to certain vegetables, explore alternatives that provide similar nutrients.

Grains: If you follow a gluten-free diet, there are various gluten-free grains available, such as quinoa, rice, and buckwheat. These grains can be used as alternatives to wheat-based products.

Proteins: If you follow a vegetarian or vegan diet, you can substitute animal-based proteins with plant-based options like legumes, tofu, tempeh, or seitan. These alternatives provide similar protein content and can be incorporated into various dishes.

Dairy and Alternatives: If you are lactose intolerant or follow a vegan diet, there are numerous dairy alternatives available, such as soy milk, almond milk, and coconut milk. These alternatives can be used in recipes or enjoyed on their own.

By exploring substitutions and alternatives, you can still meet your nutrient needs while accommodating your dietary preferences or restrictions.

Incorporating the five food groups into your meals ensures that you are consuming a wide range of nutrients necessary for optimal health. By following the balanced plate approach and making appropriate substitutions or alternatives, you can create a personalized and well-rounded diet that suits your individual needs.

Building a Balanced Plate

Building a balanced plate is an essential aspect of maintaining a healthy and nutritious diet. It involves selecting the right combination of foods from different food groups to ensure that your body receives all the necessary nutrients it needs to function optimally. By creating a balanced plate, you can promote overall well-being, support weight management, and reduce the risk of chronic diseases.

A balanced plate typically consists of a variety of foods from the five main food groups: fruits, vegetables, grains, protein, and dairy (or dairy alternatives). Each food group provides unique nutrients that contribute to your overall health. Let's explore how you can build a balanced plate by incorporating foods from each group:

Fruits:

Fruits are packed with essential vitamins, minerals, and dietary fiber. They are also a great source of natural sugars, which provide energy. When building your plate, aim to include a variety of fruits to maximize the nutritional benefits. For example, you can add sliced strawberries to your breakfast cereal, enjoy a banana as a mid-morning snack, or include a side of mixed berries with your lunch.

Vegetables:

Vegetables are rich in vitamins, minerals, and dietary fiber. They are low in calories and high in nutrients, making them an excellent addition to any balanced plate. Aim to include a variety of colorful vegetables to ensure you receive a wide range of nutrients. For example, you can have a side of steamed broccoli with your dinner, add spinach to your omelet, or enjoy a mixed salad with lunch.

Grains:

Grains provide carbohydrates, which are the body's primary source of energy. When selecting grains for your plate, opt for whole grains whenever possible. Whole grains are less processed and retain more of their natural nutrients and fiber. Examples of whole grains include brown rice, quinoa, whole wheat bread, and oats. You can include a serving of whole grains in your meals by having a side of brown rice with your stir-fry, enjoying a whole wheat sandwich for lunch, or adding oats to your breakfast smoothie.

Protein:

Protein is essential for building and repairing tissues, supporting immune function, and maintaining healthy hair, skin, and nails. There are various sources of protein, including lean meats, poultry, fish, eggs, legumes, and tofu. When building your plate, aim to include a serving of protein. For example, you can have grilled chicken breast with your dinner, enjoy a hard-boiled egg as a snack, or add black beans to your salad.

Dairy (or Dairy Alternatives):

Dairy products are a good source of calcium, which is essential for strong bones and teeth. If you consume dairy, include a serving of low-fat milk, yogurt, or cheese in your balanced plate. However, if you follow a dairy-free or vegan diet, there are plenty of dairy alternatives available, such as almond milk, soy yogurt, or tofu-based cheese. Incorporate these alternatives into your plate to ensure you meet your calcium needs.

By including foods from each of these food groups, you can create a balanced plate that provides a wide range of nutrients. However, it's important to consider portion sizes and moderation. Even though all these food groups are essential, consuming them in excessive amounts can lead to an imbalance in your diet.

To ensure portion control, you can use the "MyPlate" method as a visual guide. Imagine dividing your plate into four sections: one-half for fruits and vegetables, one-quarter for grains, and one-quarter for protein. Additionally, include a serving of dairy or dairy alternatives on the side. This method helps you visualize the appropriate proportions of each food group.

Remember, building a balanced plate is not limited to a single meal. It should be practiced throughout the day to ensure consistent nutrient intake. For example, if you have a balanced plate for breakfast, aim to continue this practice for lunch, dinner, and snacks. Consistency is key in maintaining a well-rounded diet.

Incorporating a variety of foods from different food groups not only provides essential nutrients but also adds flavor and enjoyment to your meals. Experiment with different recipes, flavors, and cooking methods to keep your meals interesting and satisfying. Building a balanced plate is a lifelong habit that can contribute to your overall health and well-being.

Sample Meal Plans for Different Food Groups

When it comes to maintaining a balanced diet, it's important to ensure that you are consuming a variety of foods from each of the five food groups. This not only provides your body with the necessary nutrients it needs to function properly, but it also helps to prevent nutrient deficiencies and promote overall health and well-being.

To help you get started on your journey to a balanced diet, here are some sample meal plans that incorporate foods from each of the five food groups:

Meal Plan 1: Breakfast

1 cup of oatmeal topped with sliced bananas and a sprinkle of cinnamon (Grains and Fruits)

1 boiled egg (Protein)

1 cup of low-fat milk (Dairy)

Meal Plan 1: Lunch

Grilled chicken breast with a side of steamed broccoli and brown rice (Protein, Vegetables, and

Grains)

Mixed green salad with cherry tomatoes, cucumbers, and a drizzle of olive oil and vinegar (Vegetables and Healthy Fats)

Meal Plan 1: Snack

1 small apple with 1 tablespoon of almond butter (Fruits and Healthy Fats)

Meal Plan 1: Dinner

Baked salmon with a side of roasted sweet potatoes and sautéed spinach (Protein, Vegetables, and Grains)

1 cup of Greek yogurt with mixed berries for dessert (Dairy and Fruits)

Meal Plan 2: Breakfast

Veggie omelet made with egg whites, spinach, tomatoes, and mushrooms (Protein and Vegetables)

1 slice of whole wheat toast (Grains)

Meal Plan 2: Lunch

Quinoa salad with mixed vegetables (such as bell peppers, carrots, and zucchini) and a lemon vinaigrette dressing (Grains and Vegetables)

1 cup of low-fat cottage cheese (Dairy)

Meal Plan 2: Snack

1 small handful of almonds (Protein and Healthy Fats)

Meal Plan 2: Dinner

Grilled lean steak with a side of roasted Brussels sprouts and quinoa (Protein, Vegetables, and Grains)

1 cup of mixed fruit for dessert (Fruits)

Meal Plan 3: Breakfast

Whole grain toast topped with avocado and a poached egg (Grains, Healthy Fats, and Protein)

1 cup of low-fat milk (Dairy)

Meal Plan 3: Lunch

Chickpea salad with mixed greens, cherry tomatoes, cucumbers, and a lemon tahini dressing (Protein, Vegetables, and Healthy Fats)

1 small orange (Fruits)

Meal Plan 3: Snack

Carrot sticks with hummus (Vegetables and Protein)

Meal Plan 3: Dinner

Grilled shrimp skewers with a side of quinoa and roasted asparagus (Protein, Grains, and Vegetables)

1 cup of low-fat yogurt with honey for dessert (Dairy)

These sample meal plans are just a starting point and can be customized to suit your individual preferences and dietary needs. Remember to include a variety of foods from each food group to ensure that you are getting all the essential nutrients your body needs.

It's also important to note that portion sizes should be adjusted based on your specific calorie needs and goals. Consulting with a registered dietitian or nutritionist can help you create a personalized meal plan that meets your unique requirements.

By incorporating these sample meal plans into your daily routine, you can take a step towards achieving a balanced diet that supports your overall health and well-being.

Food Group Substitutions and Alternatives

When it comes to following a balanced diet, it's important to have a variety of foods from each food group. However, there may be times when you need to make substitutions or find alternatives due to dietary restrictions, allergies, or personal preferences. In this section, we will explore some common food group substitutions and alternatives that can help you maintain a balanced diet while accommodating your specific needs.

Substituting Protein Sources

Protein is an essential macronutrient that plays a crucial role in building and repairing tissues, supporting immune function, and providing energy. While meat and poultry are common sources of protein, there are plenty of plant-based alternatives for those who follow a vegetarian or vegan diet or simply want to reduce their meat consumption.

Legumes: Foods like beans, lentils, and chickpeas are excellent sources of protein and can be used as a substitute for meat in dishes like chili, soups, and stews. They are also versatile and can be made into patties or used as a filling for tacos or wraps.

Tofu and Tempeh: These soy-based products are popular among vegetarians and vegans as they provide a good amount of protein. Tofu can be used in stir-fries, curries, and salads, while tempeh can be marinated and grilled or used as a substitute for ground meat in recipes like spaghetti bolognese.

Quinoa: This ancient grain is not only a great source of protein but also contains all nine essential amino acids. It can be used as a base for salads, added to soups, or used as a substitute for rice in dishes like stir-fries.

Alternatives for Dairy Products

Dairy products are a significant source of calcium, vitamin D, and protein. However, some individuals may be lactose intolerant or have dairy allergies. Fortunately, there are several alternatives available that can provide similar nutrients.

Plant-based Milk: Soy milk, almond milk, oat milk, and coconut milk are popular dairy milk alternatives. They can be used in place of regular milk in recipes, cereals, smoothies, and coffee.

Yogurt Alternatives: Coconut milk yogurt, almond milk yogurt, and soy milk yogurt are excellent alternatives for those who cannot consume dairy. They can be enjoyed on their own or used in recipes that call for yogurt.

Cheese Substitutes: There are various plant-based cheese alternatives made from nuts, soy, or tapioca starch. These alternatives can be used in sandwiches, pizzas, or pasta dishes.

Swapping Grains and Starches

Grains and starches are an essential part of a balanced diet, providing energy and essential nutrients. However, if you have gluten intolerance or follow a low-carb diet, you may need to find suitable alternatives.

Gluten-Free Grains: Quinoa, rice, corn, millet, and buckwheat are gluten-free grains that can be used as substitutes for wheat-based products like bread, pasta, and flour.

Cauliflower Rice: For those following a low-carb or keto diet, cauliflower rice is an excellent alternative to traditional rice. It can be used in stir-fries, fried rice, or as a base for grain-free salads.

Sweet Potato or Zucchini Noodles: Instead of traditional pasta, spiralized sweet potatoes or zucchini can be used to create delicious and nutritious noodle dishes. They can be enjoyed with various sauces and toppings.

Fruit and Vegetable Substitutions

Fruits and vegetables are vital sources of vitamins, minerals, and fiber. However, if you have allergies or simply want to try something different, there are alternatives available.

Seasonal Fruits and Vegetables: Instead of relying on the same fruits and vegetables year-round, try incorporating seasonal produce into your diet. This not only provides variety but also ensures that you are consuming fresh and locally sourced foods.

Frozen Fruits and Vegetables: If fresh produce is not readily available or you want to stock up on certain items, frozen fruits and vegetables are a convenient and nutritious alternative. They are often flash-frozen at their peak ripeness, preserving their nutrients.

Vegetable Noodles: Spiralized vegetables like zucchini, carrots, or beets can be used as a substitute for traditional pasta. They can be enjoyed raw in salads or lightly cooked in stir-fries.

Healthy Fat Alternatives

While fats should be consumed in moderation, they are an essential part of a balanced diet. However, not all fats are created equal, and it's important to choose healthier alternatives when possible.

Avocado: Instead of using butter or mayonnaise on sandwiches or toast, try spreading mashed avocado. Avocado is rich in heart-healthy monounsaturated fats and provides a creamy texture.

Nuts and Seeds: Instead of using butter or oil in cooking or baking, consider using ground nuts or seeds like almonds, walnuts, or flaxseeds. They add flavor, texture, and healthy fats to your dishes.

Olive Oil: Swap out unhealthy oils like vegetable or canola oil with extra virgin olive oil. It is rich in monounsaturated fats and has been associated with numerous health benefits.

Remember, while substitutions and alternatives can be helpful, it's essential to ensure that you are still meeting your nutritional needs. Consult with a healthcare professional or registered dietitian to ensure that your dietary choices align with your specific requirements.

HYDRATION AND ITS IMPORTANCE

The Role of Water in the Body

Water is an essential component of our bodies, playing a crucial role in maintaining overall health and well-being. It is often referred to as the "elixir of life" due to its vital functions and the numerous benefits it provides. In this section, we will explore the importance of water in the body and how it contributes to our overall health.

The Importance of Water

Water is the most abundant substance in our bodies, making up about 60% of our total body weight. It is involved in almost every bodily function and is essential for the proper functioning of various organs and systems. Here are some key roles that water plays in the body:

Hydration: Water is the primary component of bodily fluids, including blood, lymph, and digestive juices. It helps transport nutrients, oxygen, and waste products throughout the body, ensuring the proper functioning of cells and organs.

Temperature Regulation: Water helps regulate body temperature through processes like sweating and evaporation. When we sweat, water on the skin's surface evaporates, cooling down the body and preventing overheating.

Digestion and Nutrient Absorption: Water is essential for the digestion and absorption of nutrients. It helps break down food, aids in the absorption of nutrients in the digestive tract, and facilitates the movement of waste through the intestines.

Joint Lubrication: Water acts as a lubricant for joints, allowing smooth movement and reducing friction between bones. It helps cushion and protect the joints, preventing discomfort and promoting flexibility.

Cognitive Function: Proper hydration is crucial for optimal brain function. Dehydration can impair cognitive abilities, including concentration, alertness, and short-term memory. Drinking enough water can help improve mental clarity and focus.

Kidney Function: Water plays a vital role in maintaining kidney health. It helps flush out waste products and toxins from the body through urine. Sufficient water intake can reduce the risk of kidney stones and urinary tract infections.

Skin Health: Adequate hydration is essential for maintaining healthy skin. Water helps moisturize the skin, improve elasticity, and promote a youthful appearance. It also aids in the removal of toxins, reducing the risk of skin problems like acne and dryness.

How Much Water Should You Drink?

The amount of water each person needs can vary depending on various factors, including age, sex, activity level, and overall health. While there is no one-size-fits-all recommendation, a general guideline is to drink at least eight 8-ounce glasses of water per day, which is equivalent to about 2 liters or half a gallon.

However, individual water needs may differ. Some factors that can influence water requirements include:

Activity Level: Physical activity increases fluid loss through sweat, so individuals who engage in regular exercise or have a physically demanding job may need to drink more water to stay adequately hydrated.

Climate and Environment: Hot and humid climates can lead to increased sweating and fluid loss, requiring higher water intake. Similarly, high altitudes and dry environments can also increase water needs.

Health Conditions: Certain medical conditions, such as kidney stones or urinary tract infections, may require increased water intake as part of the treatment plan. It's important to consult with a healthcare professional for personalized recommendations.

Pregnancy and Breastfeeding: Pregnant and breastfeeding women have higher water needs to support the growth and development of the fetus or infant. It is recommended for them to drink additional fluids to stay hydrated.

To ensure adequate hydration, it's important to listen to your body's signals and drink water whenever you feel thirsty. Additionally, monitoring the color of your urine can provide a good indication of hydration status. Clear or pale yellow urine generally indicates proper hydration, while dark yellow or amber-colored urine may suggest dehydration.

Staying Hydrated Throughout the Day

Drinking enough water throughout the day is essential for maintaining optimal hydration. Here are some tips to help you stay hydrated:

Carry a Water Bottle: Keep a reusable water bottle with you wherever you go. This will serve as a reminder to drink water regularly and make it easily accessible.

Set Reminders: Use alarms or smartphone apps to remind yourself to drink water at regular intervals. This can be especially helpful if you tend to forget to hydrate throughout the day.

Infuse Your Water: If you find plain water boring, try infusing it with fruits, herbs, or vegetables to add flavor. Examples include adding slices of lemon, cucumber, or mint leaves to your water bottle.

Eat Hydrating Foods: Many fruits and vegetables have high water content and can contribute to your overall hydration. Examples include watermelon, cucumbers, oranges, and strawberries.

Drink Before, During, and After Exercise: Hydrate before, during, and after physical activity to replenish fluids lost through sweat. Sip on water or a sports drink to maintain hydration during prolonged or intense exercise.

Limit Caffeine and Alcohol: Caffeine and alcohol can have a diuretic effect, increasing fluid loss. While moderate consumption is generally fine, it's important to balance it with adequate water intake.

Remember, thirst is not always a reliable indicator of hydration. By the time you feel thirsty, you may already be mildly dehydrated. Therefore, it's important to make a conscious effort to drink water regularly throughout the day.

Hydration Tips for Exercise and Physical Activity

Proper hydration is particularly important during exercise and physical activity. When you're active, your body loses more water through sweat, and adequate fluid intake becomes crucial. Here are some hydration tips to keep in mind:

Pre-Exercise Hydration: Drink about 16-20 ounces (500-600 ml) of water 2-3 hours before exercise to ensure adequate hydration. If you're exercising first thing in the morning, start your day with a glass of water.

During Exercise Hydration: Drink water or a sports drink every 15-20 minutes during exercise, especially if it lasts longer than 60 minutes or if you're exercising in hot or humid conditions. Aim to consume about 7-10 ounces (200-300 ml) of fluid every 10-20 minutes.

Post-Exercise Hydration: Replenish fluids after exercise by drinking water or a sports drink. Aim to drink at least 16-24 ounces (500-750 ml) of fluid for every pound (0.5 kg) of body weight lost during exercise.

Consider Electrolyte Replacement: During prolonged or intense exercise, especially in hot conditions, you may need to replace electrolytes lost through sweat. Sports drinks or electrolyte-enhanced water can help replenish these minerals.

Listen to Your Body: Pay attention to signs of dehydration during exercise, such as excessive thirst, dizziness, fatigue, or dark-colored urine. If you experience any of these symptoms, take a break, hydrate, and seek shade if necessary.

Remember that individual hydration needs can vary based on factors like body size, sweat rate, and exercise intensity. It's important to experiment and find what works best for you. If you have specific concerns or medical conditions, consult with a healthcare professional or a registered dietitian for personalized hydration recommendations.

In conclusion, water is an essential nutrient that plays a vital role in maintaining overall health and well-being. It is involved in numerous bodily functions and is necessary for optimal organ and system functioning. By understanding the importance of water and staying adequately hydrated, you can support your body's optimal performance and promote overall health.

How Much Water Should You Drink?

Water is an essential component of our bodies, making up about 60% of our total body weight. It plays a crucial role in maintaining various bodily functions, including temperature regulation, digestion, nutrient absorption, and waste removal. Staying hydrated is vital for overall health and well-being. But how much water should you drink? The answer to this question depends on several factors, including your age, sex, activity level, and overall health.

Factors Affecting Water Needs

The amount of water you need to drink can vary based on several factors. Here are some key factors that influence your water requirements:

Age: Infants and children have higher water needs compared to adults due to their higher metabolic rate and greater water loss through activities like sweating and breathing. Older adults may also have increased water needs due to changes in kidney function and decreased thirst sensation.

Sex: Men generally have higher water needs than women due to their larger body size and higher muscle mass. However, women's water needs may increase during pregnancy and breastfeeding.

Activity Level: Physical activity and exercise increase water loss through sweat. If you engage in intense workouts or live an active lifestyle, you will need to drink more water to compensate for the fluid loss.

Climate and Environment: Hot and humid climates can lead to increased sweating and higher water needs. Similarly, high altitudes and dry environments can also increase water loss through respiration.

Health Conditions: Certain health conditions, such as fever, diarrhea, and vomiting, can cause excessive fluid loss and increase your water requirements. Additionally, individuals with specific medical conditions, like kidney stones or urinary tract infections, may need to drink more water to prevent complications.

General Guidelines for Water Intake

While individual water needs can vary, there are some general guidelines you can follow to ensure adequate hydration:

The 8x8 Rule: This rule suggests drinking eight 8-ounce glasses of water per day, which is equivalent to about 2 liters or half a gallon. While this guideline is easy to remember, it may not be suitable for everyone, especially those with higher water needs.

The Institute of Medicine (IOM) Recommendations: The IOM recommends a daily water intake of about 3.7 liters (or about 13 cups) for men and 2.7 liters (or about 9 cups) for women. These recommendations include water from all sources, including beverages and food.

Thirst and Urine Color: Pay attention to your body's thirst signals and the color of your urine. Thirst is a reliable indicator that your body needs more water. Additionally, clear or light-colored urine indicates adequate hydration, while dark-colored urine may be a sign of dehydration.

Activity-Related Hydration: If you engage in physical activity or exercise, it's essential to drink water before, during, and after your workout to replace the fluids lost through sweat. The American College of Sports Medicine recommends drinking about 16-20 ounces of water 2-3 hours before exercise and 8-10 ounces every 10-20 minutes during exercise.

Individual Needs: Remember that individual water needs can vary, so it's essential to listen to your body and adjust your water intake accordingly. Factors such as body weight, sweat rate, and overall health should be considered when determining your specific water requirements.

Tips for Staying Hydrated

In addition to knowing how much water to drink, here are some practical tips to help you stay hydrated throughout the day:

Carry a Water Bottle: Keep a reusable water bottle with you at all times, whether you're at work, running errands, or exercising. Having water readily available will remind you to drink and make it easier to meet your hydration goals.

Set Reminders: If you struggle to remember to drink water, set reminders on your phone or use apps that send notifications to prompt you to hydrate regularly.

Infuse Your Water: If you find plain water boring, infuse it with fruits, herbs, or vegetables to add flavor and make it more enjoyable. Try combinations like lemon and mint, cucumber and lime, or strawberry and basil.

Eat Hydrating Foods: Many fruits and vegetables have high water content and can contribute to your overall hydration. Include foods like watermelon, cucumbers, oranges, and strawberries in your diet to increase your water intake.

Monitor Your Urine: Keep an eye on the color of your urine throughout the day. If it's pale yellow or clear, you're likely well-hydrated. If it's dark yellow or amber, it's a sign that you need to drink more water.

Remember that water is the best choice for hydration, but other beverages like herbal tea, unsweetened coffee, and milk can also contribute to your daily fluid intake. However, be mindful of sugary drinks and caffeinated beverages, as they can have diuretic effects and may not be as hydrating as plain water.

By understanding your individual water needs and following these tips, you can ensure that you stay adequately hydrated and support your overall health and well-being.

Staying Hydrated Throughout the Day

Staying hydrated is essential for maintaining optimal health and well-being. Water plays a crucial role in various bodily functions, including regulating body temperature, aiding digestion, transporting nutrients, and flushing out waste products. It is important to ensure that you are adequately hydrated throughout the day to support these functions and promote overall health.

Importance of Hydration

Proper hydration is vital for maintaining the balance of bodily fluids. Water makes up a significant portion of our body weight and is involved in numerous physiological processes. When you are dehydrated, your body may struggle to perform these functions efficiently, leading to various health issues.

One of the primary functions of water is regulating body temperature. When you are active or exposed to hot weather, your body sweats to cool down. Sweating helps dissipate heat, but it also leads to fluid loss. By staying hydrated, you can replenish the lost fluids and prevent dehydration, which can cause fatigue, dizziness, and even heatstroke.

Water also plays a crucial role in digestion. It helps break down food, absorb nutrients, and eliminate waste products. Insufficient hydration can lead to digestive problems such as constipation and indigestion. By drinking enough water, you can support proper digestion and maintain a healthy digestive system.

Furthermore, water is essential for transporting nutrients throughout the body. It acts as a medium for delivering nutrients to cells and removing waste products. Without adequate hydration, this process may be compromised, affecting the overall functioning of your body.

Signs of Dehydration

It is important to be aware of the signs of dehydration so that you can take prompt action to rehydrate. Some common signs of dehydration include:

Thirst: Feeling thirsty is one of the first signs that your body needs water. It is important not to ignore this signal and drink water as soon as you feel thirsty.

Dark-colored urine: Urine color can indicate your hydration status. If your urine is dark yellow or amber, it may be a sign of dehydration. Ideally, your urine should be pale yellow or clear.

Dry mouth and lips: When you are dehydrated, your mouth and lips may feel dry and parched. Drinking water can help alleviate this symptom.

Fatigue and dizziness: Dehydration can cause fatigue, dizziness, and a lack of energy. If you are feeling tired or lightheaded, it may be a sign that you need to hydrate.

Headaches: Dehydration can trigger headaches and migraines. Drinking water can help relieve these symptoms.

Tips for Staying Hydrated

To ensure that you stay hydrated throughout the day, consider implementing the following tips:

Carry a water bottle: Keep a reusable water bottle with you at all times. This will serve as a reminder to drink water regularly and make it easily accessible.

Set reminders: Use alarms or smartphone apps to remind yourself to drink water at regular intervals. This can be especially helpful if you tend to forget to hydrate.

Drink water with meals: Make it a habit to drink a glass of water with each meal. This not only helps with hydration but also aids digestion.

Flavor your water: If you find plain water boring, try infusing it with fruits, herbs, or cucumber slices to add a refreshing flavor. This can make drinking water more enjoyable and encourage you to consume more.

Eat hydrating foods: Many fruits and vegetables have high water content and can contribute to your overall hydration. Include foods like watermelon, cucumbers, oranges, and strawberries in your diet.

Monitor your urine color: Pay attention to the color of your urine. If it is pale yellow or clear, it indicates that you are adequately hydrated. Dark-colored urine may be a sign that you need to drink more water.

Limit caffeine and alcohol intake: Both caffeine and alcohol can have a diuretic effect, increasing fluid loss from the body. If you consume these beverages, make sure to balance them with an adequate intake of water.

Drink water before, during, and after exercise: When you engage in physical activity, your body loses water through sweat. Drink water before, during, and after exercise to replenish the lost fluids and maintain hydration.

Keep water visible: Place a glass or bottle of water on your desk, kitchen counter, or bedside table as a visual reminder to drink water throughout the day.

Listen to your body: Pay attention to your body's signals and drink water when you feel thirsty. Thirst is a natural mechanism that indicates your body's need for hydration.

By incorporating these tips into your daily routine, you can ensure that you stay adequately hydrated and support your overall health and well-being. Remember, maintaining proper hydration is a simple yet crucial aspect of a balanced diet.

Hydration Tips for Exercise and Physical Activity

Staying properly hydrated is essential for overall health and well-being, especially when engaging in exercise and physical activity. When we exercise, our bodies lose water through sweat, and it's crucial to replenish those fluids to maintain optimal performance and prevent dehydration. In this section, we will explore some hydration tips specifically tailored for exercise and physical activity.

Importance of Hydration during Exercise

During exercise, our bodies generate heat, causing an increase in body temperature. To regulate this temperature, we sweat, which leads to fluid loss. If we don't replace these lost fluids, we can become dehydrated, which can negatively impact our performance and even our health.

Proper hydration during exercise offers several benefits:

Optimal Performance: When adequately hydrated, our bodies can perform at their best. Hydration helps maintain blood volume, which is essential for delivering oxygen and nutrients to our muscles.

It also helps remove waste products, such as lactic acid, which can cause muscle fatigue.

Temperature Regulation: Sweating is our body's natural cooling mechanism. By staying hydrated, we support this process, helping to regulate our body temperature and prevent overheating.

Energy Levels: Dehydration can lead to feelings of fatigue and decreased energy levels. By staying hydrated, we can maintain our energy levels and sustain our exercise routine for longer durations.

Joint Lubrication: Hydration plays a vital role in maintaining the lubrication of our joints. This is particularly important for activities that involve impact or repetitive movements, such as running or jumping.

Hydration Tips for Exercise and Physical Activity

To ensure proper hydration during exercise and physical activity, consider the following tips:

Pre-Hydration: Start your exercise session well-hydrated by drinking fluids throughout the day leading up to your workout. Aim to consume around 16-20 ounces (473-591 ml) of water or a sports drink 2-3 hours before exercising.

During Exercise: During your workout, it's essential to replace the fluids you lose through sweat. The American College of Sports Medicine recommends drinking 7-10 ounces (207-296 ml) of fluid every 10-20 minutes during exercise. If you're engaging in intense or prolonged exercise, consider a sports drink that contains electrolytes to replenish both fluids and essential minerals.

Post-Exercise Hydration: After your workout, continue to hydrate to replace any remaining fluid losses. Aim to drink at least 16-24 ounces (473-710 ml) of fluid for every pound (0.45 kg) of body weight lost during exercise.

Monitor Urine Color: One way to gauge your hydration status is by monitoring the color of your urine. Ideally, your urine should be pale yellow or straw-colored. Darker urine may indicate dehydration, while clear urine may suggest overhydration.

Hydration and Electrolytes: When we sweat, we not only lose water but also essential electrolytes like sodium, potassium, and magnesium. If you're engaging in prolonged or intense exercise lasting more than an hour, consider consuming a sports drink or electrolyte-rich fluids to replenish these electrolytes.

Individual Hydration Needs: Remember that everyone's hydration needs may vary based on factors such as body weight, exercise intensity, duration, and environmental conditions. It's essential to listen to your body and adjust your fluid intake accordingly.

Hydration Beyond Water: While water is an excellent choice for hydration, other fluids can also contribute to your overall fluid intake. For example, low-fat milk, herbal teas, and 100% fruit juices can provide hydration along with additional nutrients.

Hydration and Weather Conditions: Be mindful of the environmental conditions when exercising outdoors. In hot and humid weather, you may need to increase your fluid intake to compensate for increased sweating and higher fluid losses.

Hydration and Intense Exercise: If you're engaging in high-intensity exercise or endurance activities, it may be beneficial to consume carbohydrates along with fluids. This can help provide energy and maintain performance levels during prolonged exercise sessions.

Listen to Your Body: Pay attention to your body's signals of thirst and fatigue. If you feel thirsty, it's a sign that you're already partially dehydrated. Drink fluids regularly, even if you don't feel thirsty, to stay ahead of dehydration.

Remember, staying hydrated is not only important during exercise but also throughout the day. Make it a habit to drink fluids regularly, even when you're not physically active. By maintaining proper hydration, you can support your overall health and optimize your exercise performance

BALANCING MACRONUTRIENTS

Understanding Carbohydrates, Proteins, and Fats

In order to achieve a balanced diet, it is important to understand the role of macronutrients in our body. Macronutrients are the nutrients that our body needs in large quantities to function properly. The three main macronutrients are carbohydrates, proteins, and fats. Each of these macronutrients plays a unique role in our body and provides us with the energy and essential nutrients we need to thrive.

Carbohydrates

Carbohydrates are the body's primary source of energy. They are found in a variety of foods such as grains, fruits, vegetables, and legumes. Carbohydrates are made up of sugar molecules, which are broken down by our body into glucose, the main source of fuel for our cells.

There are two types of carbohydrates: simple carbohydrates and complex carbohydrates. Simple carbohydrates, also known as sugars, are found in foods like candy, soda, and baked goods. They provide quick energy but lack essential nutrients. On the other hand, complex carbohydrates, found in foods like whole grains, beans, and vegetables, provide a steady release of energy and are rich in fiber, vitamins, and minerals.

It is important to choose complex carbohydrates over simple carbohydrates as they provide sustained energy and are more nutritious. Examples of complex carbohydrates include whole wheat bread, brown rice, quinoa, and sweet potatoes.

Proteins

Proteins are essential for the growth, repair, and maintenance of our body tissues. They are made up of amino acids, which are the building blocks of proteins. Our body needs 20 different amino acids to function properly, and while our body can produce some of these amino acids, there are nine essential amino acids that we must obtain from our diet.

Protein-rich foods include meat, poultry, fish, eggs, dairy products, legumes, nuts, and seeds. Animal sources of protein, such as meat and dairy, provide all nine essential amino acids, making them complete proteins. Plant-based sources of protein, such as legumes and grains, may lack one or more essential amino acids, but can be combined to form complete proteins.

It is important to include a variety of protein sources in our diet to ensure we are getting all the essential amino acids. For example, a meal that combines beans and rice or peanut butter on whole wheat bread can provide a complete protein.

Fats

Fats are an essential part of a balanced diet and play a crucial role in our body. They provide energy, help absorb fat-soluble vitamins, protect our organs, and insulate our body. However, not all fats are created equal. There are different types of fats, including saturated fats, trans fats, monounsaturated fats, and polyunsaturated fats.

Saturated fats, found in foods like butter, red meat, and full-fat dairy products, should be consumed in moderation as they can increase the risk of heart disease. Trans fats, found in processed foods, fried foods, and baked goods, should be avoided as they are the unhealthiest type of fat.

On the other hand, monounsaturated fats and polyunsaturated fats are considered healthy fats. They can be found in foods like avocados, olive oil, nuts, and fatty fish. These fats can help lower bad cholesterol levels and reduce the risk of heart disease.

It is important to include healthy fats in our diet while limiting the intake of unhealthy fats. For example, instead of frying foods in butter or vegetable oil, we can use olive oil or avocado oil. Instead of snacking on chips or cookies, we can opt for a handful of nuts or seeds.

Understanding the role of carbohydrates, proteins, and fats in our body is essential for achieving a balanced diet. By choosing the right sources and proportions of these macronutrients, we can provide our body with the energy and nutrients it needs to function optimally. Remember to focus on whole, unprocessed foods and make mindful choices to support your overall health and well-being.

The Role of Each Macronutrient in the Body

Macronutrients are the essential nutrients that our bodies need in large quantities to function properly. They include carbohydrates, proteins, and fats. Each macronutrient plays a unique role in the body, providing energy, supporting growth and repair, and maintaining overall health. Understanding the role of each macronutrient is crucial for achieving a balanced diet and optimizing our well-being.

Carbohydrates

Carbohydrates are the body's primary source of energy. They are broken down into glucose, which is used by our cells to fuel various bodily functions. Carbohydrates can be found in a wide range of foods, including grains, fruits, vegetables, legumes, and dairy products. They come in two forms: simple and complex carbohydrates.

Simple carbohydrates, also known as sugars, are quickly digested and provide a rapid burst of energy. Examples include table sugar, honey, and fruit juices. While they can be enjoyed in moderation, it's important to limit our intake of added sugars, as they can contribute to weight gain and increase the risk of chronic diseases.

Complex carbohydrates, on the other hand, are digested more slowly, providing a steady release of energy. They are rich in fiber, vitamins, and minerals, and can be found in foods like whole grains, vegetables, and legumes. These carbohydrates are an essential part of a balanced diet, as they promote satiety, support digestive health, and help regulate blood sugar levels.

Proteins

Proteins are the building blocks of our body. They are responsible for the growth, repair, and maintenance of tissues, organs, and cells. Proteins are made up of amino acids, which are essential for various physiological processes. While our bodies can produce some amino acids, there are nine essential amino acids that we must obtain from our diet.

Protein-rich foods include meat, poultry, fish, eggs, dairy products, legumes, nuts, and seeds. It's important to consume a variety of protein sources to ensure an adequate intake of all essential amino acids. Additionally, plant-based proteins can be combined to create complete protein sources, such as beans and rice or peanut butter on whole wheat bread.

Proteins also play a crucial role in hormone production, immune function, and enzyme activity. They are particularly important during periods of growth, such as childhood and adolescence, as well as during pregnancy and breastfeeding. Including lean sources of protein in our meals and snacks can help promote satiety, support muscle development, and aid in weight management.

Fats

Fats often get a bad reputation, but they are an essential part of a balanced diet. They provide energy, support cell growth, protect organs, and help the body absorb certain vitamins. However, not all fats are created equal. It's important to focus on consuming healthy fats while limiting unhealthy fats.

Healthy fats include monounsaturated and polyunsaturated fats, which can be found in foods like avocados, nuts, seeds, and fatty fish. These fats have been shown to reduce the risk of heart disease and improve cholesterol levels. They also provide essential fatty acids, such as omega-3 and omega-6, which are important for brain function and overall health.

Unhealthy fats, such as saturated and trans fats, should be limited in our diet. These fats can raise cholesterol levels and increase the risk of heart disease. They are commonly found in processed foods, fried foods, and high-fat dairy products. Reading food labels and choosing products low in saturated and trans fats can help promote heart health.

It's important to note that fats are high in calories, so portion control is key. Incorporating healthy fats into our meals, such as using olive oil in cooking or adding avocado to a salad, can help us feel satisfied and support overall well-being.

In conclusion, each macronutrient plays a vital role in our body's functioning. Carbohydrates provide energy, proteins support growth and repair, and fats provide essential nutrients and protect our organs. By understanding the role of each macronutrient and incorporating them into a balanced diet, we can optimize our health and well-being. Remember to choose whole food sources and practice portion control to maintain a healthy balance.

Balancing Macronutrients for Optimal Health

Balancing macronutrients is an essential aspect of maintaining optimal health. Macronutrients, which include carbohydrates, proteins, and fats, are the primary sources of energy for our bodies. Each macronutrient plays a unique role in our overall well-being, and finding the right balance between them is crucial for achieving and sustaining good health.

The Importance of Balancing Macronutrients

When it comes to our diet, the proportions of macronutrients we consume can significantly impact our health. A well-balanced intake of carbohydrates, proteins, and fats ensures that our bodies receive the necessary nutrients to function optimally. Here's a closer look at the role of each macronutrient and how to strike the right balance:

Carbohydrates

Carbohydrates are the body's primary source of energy. They provide fuel for our muscles, brain, and other organs. However, not all carbohydrates are created equal. It's important to focus on consuming complex carbohydrates, such as whole grains, legumes, and vegetables, which provide a steady release of energy and are rich in fiber. Simple carbohydrates, found in sugary snacks and processed foods, can lead to energy spikes and crashes. Strive to include a variety of complex carbohydrates in your diet to maintain stable energy levels throughout the day.

Proteins

Proteins are the building blocks of our bodies. They are essential for the growth, repair, and maintenance of tissues, muscles, and organs. Including adequate protein in your diet is crucial for supporting muscle development, immune function, and hormone production. Good sources of protein include lean meats, poultry, fish, eggs, dairy products, legumes, and plant-based sources such as tofu and tempeh. Aim to include a variety of protein sources in your meals to ensure you're getting a complete range of essential amino acids.

Fats

Contrary to popular belief, fats are an essential part of a healthy diet. They provide energy, support cell growth, protect organs, and help absorb certain vitamins. However, not all fats are created equal. Saturated and trans fats, found in fried foods, processed snacks, and fatty meats, can increase the risk of heart disease and other health issues. On the other hand, unsaturated fats, found in foods like avocados, nuts, seeds, and olive oil, are beneficial for heart health. Strive to include more unsaturated fats in your diet while limiting your intake of saturated and trans fats.

Striking the Right Balance

Finding the right balance of macronutrients can be a personal journey, as individual needs vary based on factors such as age, sex, activity level, and overall health. However, there are some general guidelines that can help you achieve a balanced macronutrient intake:

Assess Your Needs

Start by assessing your individual needs and goals. Consider factors such as your activity level, body composition goals, and any specific dietary requirements or restrictions you may have. Consulting with a registered dietitian can provide valuable insights tailored to your unique needs.

Determine Your Macronutrient Ratios

Once you have a clear understanding of your needs, you can determine the appropriate macronutrient ratios for your diet. While there is no one-size-fits-all approach, a balanced diet typically consists of approximately 45-65% of calories from carbohydrates, 10-35% from protein, and 20-35% from fats. These ranges can be adjusted based on individual preferences and goals.

Prioritize Whole Foods

Regardless of your macronutrient ratios, it's important to prioritize whole, nutrient-dense foods. Opt for whole grains, lean proteins, and healthy fats from natural sources. These foods not only provide essential macronutrients but also offer a wide range of vitamins, minerals, and antioxidants that support overall health.

Listen to Your Body

Pay attention to how different macronutrient ratios make you feel. Experiment with different proportions and observe how your energy levels, satiety, and overall well-being are affected. Remember that balance is key, and it's important to find a macronutrient ratio that works best for you.

Meal Ideas for Balanced Macronutrient Intake

Here are some meal ideas that can help you achieve a balanced macronutrient intake:

Breakfast: A bowl of oatmeal topped with fresh berries, a dollop of Greek yogurt, and a sprinkle of nuts or seeds.

Lunch: Grilled chicken or tofu with a side of quinoa or brown rice, steamed vegetables, and a drizzle of olive oil.

Snack: A handful of almonds or a piece of fruit with a tablespoon of nut butter.

Dinner: Baked salmon or roasted chickpeas with a side of roasted sweet potatoes and a mixed green salad dressed with olive oil and vinegar.

Dessert: A small serving of Greek yogurt with a drizzle of honey and a sprinkle of granola.

Remember, these are just examples, and you can customize your meals based on your preferences and dietary needs. The key is to include a variety of whole foods from each macronutrient group to ensure a well-rounded and balanced diet.

By understanding the role of each macronutrient and finding the right balance, you can optimize your health and well-being. Remember to prioritize whole, nutrient-dense foods and listen to your body's needs. With a balanced macronutrient intake, you'll be on your way to achieving and maintaining optimal health.

Meal Ideas for Balanced Macronutrient Intake

When it comes to maintaining a balanced diet, it's important to ensure that you are consuming the right proportions of macronutrients - carbohydrates, proteins, and fats. These macronutrients play a crucial role in providing energy, supporting growth and repair, and maintaining overall health. To help you achieve a balanced macronutrient intake, here are some meal ideas that incorporate a variety of nutrient-rich foods:

Breakfast:

Scrambled eggs with whole wheat toast and avocado: This breakfast option provides a good balance of protein from the eggs, healthy fats from the avocado, and carbohydrates from the whole wheat toast.

Greek yogurt with mixed berries and a sprinkle of granola: Greek yogurt is a great source of protein, while the mixed berries add natural sweetness and fiber. The granola adds a crunchy texture and some healthy fats.

Lunch:

Grilled chicken salad with mixed greens, cherry tomatoes, cucumbers, and a drizzle of olive oil and balsamic vinegar: This salad combines lean protein from the grilled chicken, a variety of vegetables for fiber and micronutrients, and healthy fats from the olive oil.

Quinoa and black bean bowl with roasted vegetables: Quinoa is a complete protein and pairs well with black beans for added protein and fiber. Roasted vegetables like bell peppers, zucchini, and sweet potatoes provide a range of vitamins and minerals.

Snacks:

Apple slices with almond butter: Apples are a good source of carbohydrates and fiber, while almond butter adds healthy fats and protein.

Greek yogurt with a handful of nuts: Greek yogurt provides protein, while nuts like almonds or walnuts offer healthy fats and a satisfying crunch.

Dinner:

Grilled salmon with steamed broccoli and quinoa: Salmon is rich in omega-3 fatty acids and protein, while broccoli adds fiber and essential vitamins. Quinoa serves as a nutritious carbohydrate source.

Stir-fried tofu with mixed vegetables and brown rice: Tofu is a great plant-based protein option, and when combined with a variety of colorful vegetables and fiber-rich brown rice, it creates a well-balanced meal.

Dessert:

Mixed berry smoothie with a scoop of protein powder: Blend together a mix of berries, a scoop of protein powder, and a liquid of your choice (such as almond milk or coconut water) for a refreshing and protein-packed dessert option.

Dark chocolate with a handful of almonds: Dark chocolate contains antioxidants and can be enjoyed in moderation. Pair it with almonds for a satisfying combination of healthy fats and protein.

Remember, these meal ideas are just examples, and you can customize them based on your personal preferences and dietary needs. The key is to include a variety of nutrient-dense foods from different food groups to ensure a well-rounded macronutrient intake.

It's also important to note that portion sizes play a role in maintaining a balanced diet. Be mindful of your portion sizes and listen to your body's hunger and fullness cues. If you have specific dietary requirements or health concerns, it's always a good idea to consult with a registered dietitian or healthcare professional for personalized guidance.

By incorporating these meal ideas into your daily routine, you can ensure that you are getting a balanced intake of macronutrients, supporting your overall health and well-being. Remember, a balanced diet is not about restriction or deprivation but rather about nourishing your body with the right nutrients in the right proportions.

FIBER AND WHOLE GRAINS, SUGARS AND ADDED SUGARS, HEALTHY FATS, MICREONUTRIENTS

The Importance of Fiber and Whole Grains

Fiber and whole grains play a crucial role in maintaining a balanced diet and promoting overall health. They are essential components of a well-rounded eating plan and offer numerous benefits for our bodies. In this section, we will explore the importance of fiber and whole grains, their impact on our health, and how to incorporate them into our daily diet.

Understanding Fiber

Fiber is a type of carbohydrate that our bodies cannot digest. It passes through our digestive system relatively intact, providing a range of health benefits. There are two types of fiber: soluble and insoluble.

Soluble fiber dissolves in water and forms a gel-like substance in our digestive tract. It helps to lower cholesterol levels, regulate blood sugar levels, and promote a feeling of fullness, which can aid in weight management. Good sources of soluble fiber include oats, barley, legumes, fruits, and vegetables.

Insoluble fiber, on the other hand, does not dissolve in water and adds bulk to our stool. It helps to prevent constipation, promote regular bowel movements, and maintain a healthy digestive system. Whole wheat products, bran, nuts, and seeds are excellent sources of insoluble fiber.

The Benefits of Fiber

Including an adequate amount of fiber in our diet offers numerous health benefits. Here are some of the key advantages of consuming fiber-rich foods:

Improved Digestive Health: Fiber promotes regular bowel movements, prevents constipation, and reduces the risk of developing digestive disorders such as diverticulitis and hemorrhoids.

Weight Management: High-fiber foods tend to be more filling, which can help control appetite and prevent overeating. Additionally, they often have fewer calories compared to low-fiber alternatives.

Heart Health: Soluble fiber helps to lower cholesterol levels by binding to cholesterol in the digestive system and preventing its absorption into the bloodstream. This, in turn, reduces the risk of heart disease and stroke.

Blood Sugar Control: Soluble fiber slows down the absorption of sugar, preventing rapid spikes in blood sugar levels. This is particularly beneficial for individuals with diabetes or those at risk of developing the condition.

Reduced Risk of Certain Cancers: A diet high in fiber, especially from whole grains and fruits, has been associated with a lower risk of colorectal cancer.

Weight Management: High-fiber foods tend to be more filling, which can help control appetite and prevent overeating. Additionally, they often have fewer calories compared to low-fiber alternatives.

Incorporating Fiber into Your Diet

Now that we understand the importance of fiber, let's explore some practical ways to incorporate it into our daily diet:

Choose Whole Grains: Opt for whole grain bread, pasta, and cereals instead of refined grains. Whole grains retain the bran and germ, which are rich in fiber and nutrients.

Include Fruits and Vegetables: Aim to consume a variety of fruits and vegetables daily. These are excellent sources of both soluble and insoluble fiber.

Snack on Nuts and Seeds: Almonds, walnuts, chia seeds, and flaxseeds are all high in fiber. Enjoy them as a snack or sprinkle them on top of salads, yogurt, or oatmeal.

Add Legumes to Your Meals: Legumes such as lentils, chickpeas, and black beans are not only rich in fiber but also provide a good source of plant-based protein. Incorporate them into soups, stews, salads, or as a meat substitute in various dishes.

Read Food Labels: When purchasing packaged foods, check the nutrition labels for the fiber content. Choose products that have a higher fiber content and avoid those that are heavily processed and low in fiber.

Gradually Increase Fiber Intake: It's important to gradually increase your fiber intake to allow your body to adjust. Sudden increases in fiber consumption can lead to digestive discomfort. Start by adding small amounts of fiber-rich foods to your meals and gradually increase over time.

The Power of Whole Grains

Whole grains are an essential part of a balanced diet and provide a wide range of nutrients, including fiber, vitamins, minerals, and antioxidants. Unlike refined grains, which have been stripped of their bran and germ, whole grains retain all parts of the grain, making them a healthier choice.

Here are some reasons why whole grains are important:

Fiber Content: Whole grains are an excellent source of dietary fiber, which aids in digestion, promotes satiety, and helps maintain a healthy weight.

Nutrient-Rich: Whole grains contain essential nutrients such as B vitamins, iron, magnesium, and selenium. These nutrients are vital for energy production, brain function, and overall well-being.

Heart Health: Consuming whole grains has been linked to a reduced risk of heart disease. The fiber, antioxidants, and phytochemicals found in whole grains contribute to improved cardiovascular health.

Blood Sugar Control: Whole grains have a lower glycemic index compared to refined grains, meaning they cause a slower and steadier rise in blood sugar levels. This is particularly beneficial for individuals with diabetes or those at risk of developing the condition.

Weight Management: Whole grains are more filling than refined grains, which can help control appetite and prevent overeating. They also tend to have a lower calorie density, making them a great choice for weight management.

Incorporating whole grains into your diet is relatively simple. Here are some tips to help you increase your whole grain intake:

Choose Whole Grain Products: Look for bread, pasta, rice, and cereals labeled as "100% whole grain" or "whole wheat." Avoid products that are labeled as "refined" or "enriched."

Experiment with Alternative Grains: Explore a variety of whole grains such as quinoa, brown rice, barley, bulgur, and farro. These grains offer unique flavors and textures and can be used in a wide range of dishes.

Start Your Day with Whole Grains: Enjoy a bowl of oatmeal or whole grain cereal for breakfast. Top it with fresh fruits, nuts, and seeds for added flavor and nutrition.

Swap Refined Grains for Whole Grains: When cooking or baking, substitute refined grains with whole grain alternatives. For example, use whole wheat flour instead of white flour in your recipes.

Snack on Whole Grain Foods: Choose whole grain crackers, popcorn, or granola bars as healthy snack options.

By incorporating fiber-rich foods and whole grains into our diet, we can reap the numerous health benefits they offer. Remember to gradually increase your fiber intake and choose whole grain options whenever possible. With these simple changes, you can enhance your overall well-being and maintain a balanced diet.

Identifying and Reducing Added Sugars

Added sugars are sugars that are added to food and beverages during processing or preparation. These sugars are not naturally present in the food and can contribute to excess calorie intake without providing any essential nutrients. Consuming too much added sugar has been linked to various health problems, including obesity, type 2 diabetes, heart disease, and tooth decay. Therefore, it is important to identify and reduce added sugars in our diet to maintain a balanced and healthy eating pattern.

Understanding Added Sugars

Added sugars can be found in a wide range of foods and beverages, including sodas, candies, baked goods, fruit drinks, flavored yogurts, and cereals. They can be listed on food labels under various names, such as sucrose, high-fructose corn syrup, corn syrup, maltose, dextrose, and fruit juice concentrates. It is essential to read food labels carefully to identify the presence of added sugars in the products we consume.

The Impact of Added Sugars on Health

Consuming excessive amounts of added sugars can lead to weight gain and obesity. These sugars provide empty calories, meaning they contribute to calorie intake without providing any beneficial nutrients. When we consume foods high in added sugars, our bodies quickly absorb the sugars, causing a rapid increase in blood sugar levels. This spike in blood sugar is followed by a crash, leading to feelings of fatigue and hunger, which can result in overeating and weight gain.

Furthermore, a high intake of added sugars has been linked to an increased risk of developing type 2 diabetes. When we consume large amounts of added sugars, our bodies may become resistant to insulin, a hormone that helps regulate blood sugar levels. Over time, this insulin resistance can lead to the development of type 2 diabetes.

Excessive consumption of added sugars can also have a negative impact on heart health. Diets high in added sugars have been associated with an increased risk of heart disease, including high blood pressure, high cholesterol levels, and inflammation. Additionally, a diet high in added sugars can contribute to tooth decay and cavities, as the sugars provide a food source for harmful bacteria in the mouth.

Strategies for Reducing Added Sugars

Reducing added sugars in our diet can be challenging, as they are often present in many processed and packaged foods. However, with some mindful choices and simple strategies, we can gradually reduce our intake of added sugars and improve our overall health. Here are some tips to help identify and reduce added sugars:

Read Food Labels: When grocery shopping, carefully read the ingredient list and nutrition facts panel on food labels. Look for products that have little to no added sugars or choose those with natural sweeteners like honey or maple syrup.

Choose Whole Foods: Opt for whole, unprocessed foods whenever possible. Fresh fruits, vegetables, lean proteins, and whole grains are naturally low in added sugars and provide essential nutrients.

Limit Sugary Beverages: Sugary drinks like sodas, fruit juices, and sweetened teas are major sources of added sugars. Instead, choose water, unsweetened tea, or infused water with fresh fruits for a refreshing and hydrating option.

Be Mindful of Hidden Sugars: Many processed foods, such as sauces, condiments, and salad dressings, contain hidden sugars. Check the labels and choose options with no added sugars or make your own at home using natural ingredients.

Reduce Sweetened Snacks: Snack foods like cookies, cakes, and candies are often high in added sugars. Opt for healthier alternatives like fresh fruit, nuts, or homemade snacks made with natural sweeteners.

Cook at Home: By preparing meals at home, you have control over the ingredients and can reduce the amount of added sugars in your dishes. Experiment with herbs, spices, and natural sweeteners like cinnamon or vanilla extract to enhance the flavor of your meals.

Practice Moderation: While it's important to reduce added sugars, it's also essential to practice moderation. Enjoying an occasional sweet treat is fine, as long as it is part of an overall balanced diet.

By being mindful of the foods we consume and making conscious choices to reduce added sugars, we can improve our overall health and well-being. Remember, small changes over time can lead to significant improvements in our diet and lifestyle.

Choosing Healthy Fats for a Balanced Diet

When it comes to maintaining a balanced diet, it's important to understand that not all fats are created equal. While fats have long been demonized as the enemy of a healthy diet, the truth is that our bodies need certain types of fats to function properly. In fact, healthy fats play a crucial role in supporting brain health, hormone production, and nutrient absorption. The key is to choose the right types of fats and consume them in moderation.

Understanding Different Types of Fats

To make informed choices about the fats you consume, it's essential to understand the different types of fats and their effects on your health. There are four main types of dietary fats:

Saturated Fats: These fats are typically solid at room temperature and are commonly found in animal products such as meat, butter, and full-fat dairy. While saturated fats have been associated with an increased risk of heart disease, recent research suggests that the link may not be as strong as once believed. However, it's still important to consume saturated fats in moderation and opt for leaner sources of protein.

Trans Fats: Trans fats are artificially created fats that are formed through a process called hydrogenation. They are commonly found in processed foods, fried foods, and baked goods. Trans fats have been shown to raise bad cholesterol levels and increase the risk of heart disease. It's best to avoid trans fats altogether by reading food labels and opting for whole, unprocessed foods.

Monounsaturated Fats: These fats are liquid at room temperature and are found in foods such as olive oil, avocados, and nuts. Monounsaturated fats have been shown to improve heart health by reducing bad cholesterol levels and increasing good cholesterol levels. They are a healthy choice when consumed in moderation.

Polyunsaturated Fats: Polyunsaturated fats are also liquid at room temperature and can be found in foods such as fatty fish, walnuts, and flaxseeds. These fats are rich in omega-3 and omega-6 fatty acids, which are essential for brain function and reducing inflammation in the body. Including polyunsaturated fats in your diet can help support heart health and overall well-being.

Incorporating Healthy Fats into Your Diet

Now that you understand the different types of fats, it's time to learn how to incorporate healthy fats into your balanced diet. Here are some practical tips to help you make healthier fat choices:

Choose Plant-Based Oils: Opt for cooking oils that are high in monounsaturated or polyunsaturated fats, such as olive oil, avocado oil, or canola oil. These oils are healthier alternatives to saturated fats and can be used for sautéing, roasting, or dressing salads.

Include Fatty Fish: Fatty fish like salmon, mackerel, and sardines are excellent sources of omega-3 fatty acids. Aim to include these fish in your diet at least twice a week to reap the benefits of their heart-healthy fats.

Snack on Nuts and Seeds: Almonds, walnuts, chia seeds, and flaxseeds are all great sources of healthy fats. They make for satisfying snacks and can be added to salads, yogurt, or smoothies for an extra nutritional boost.

Choose Lean Protein Sources: When consuming animal products, opt for lean cuts of meat and poultry, and choose low-fat dairy options. Trim visible fat from meat and remove the skin from poultry to reduce your intake of saturated fats.

Read Food Labels: When purchasing packaged foods, read the nutrition labels carefully. Look for products that are low in saturated fats and trans fats. Be aware that food manufacturers may use alternative names for trans fats, such as "partially hydrogenated oils," so it's important to be vigilant.

Moderation is Key: While healthy fats are an essential part of a balanced diet, it's important to consume them in moderation. Fats are calorie-dense, so be mindful of portion sizes to avoid excessive calorie intake.

Balancing Fats with Other Nutrients

In addition to choosing healthy fats, it's crucial to balance your fat intake with other essential nutrients. Remember that a balanced diet consists of a combination of macronutrients (carbohydrates, proteins, and fats) and micronutrients (vitamins and minerals). Here are some tips to help you achieve a well-rounded diet:

Include a Variety of Foods: To ensure you're getting a wide range of nutrients, aim to include a variety of fruits, vegetables, whole grains, lean proteins, and healthy fats in your meals.

Focus on Whole Foods: Whole foods, such as fruits, vegetables, whole grains, and lean proteins, provide a natural balance of nutrients. Processed foods, on the other hand, often contain unhealthy fats, added sugars, and excessive sodium.

Pay Attention to Portion Sizes: Even healthy fats should be consumed in moderation. Be mindful of portion sizes and avoid overindulging in high-fat foods.

Consult a Registered Dietitian: If you're unsure about how to balance your fat intake with other nutrients, consider consulting a registered dietitian. They can provide personalized guidance based on your specific dietary needs and goals.

By choosing healthy fats and balancing them with other essential nutrients, you can create a well-rounded and balanced diet that supports your overall health and well-being. Remember, it's all about making informed choices and finding the right balance for your individual needs.

Micronutrients

Micronutrients are essential nutrients that our bodies need in small amounts to function properly. Unlike macronutrients, which are required in larger quantities, micronutrients are needed in trace amounts but play a crucial role in maintaining overall health and well-being. Micronutrients include vitamins and minerals, which are found in a variety of foods and are necessary for various bodily functions.

Importance of Micronutrients

Micronutrients are involved in numerous physiological processes, including metabolism, growth, development, and immune function. They act as cofactors for enzymes, which are essential for the proper functioning of biochemical reactions in the body. Without an adequate intake of micronutrients, these processes can be compromised, leading to various health issues.

Vitamins are organic compounds that are required in small amounts for normal growth and development. They are classified into two categories: fat-soluble vitamins (A, D, E, and K) and water-soluble vitamins (B vitamins and vitamin C). Each vitamin has specific functions and plays a vital role in maintaining different aspects of health.

Minerals, on the other hand, are inorganic substances that are essential for various physiological processes. They include macrominerals, such as calcium, phosphorus, magnesium, sodium, potassium, and chloride, which are required in larger amounts, as well as trace minerals, such as iron, zinc, copper, iodine, selenium, and manganese, which are needed in smaller quantities.

Functions of Micronutrients

Micronutrients have diverse functions in the body, and each vitamin and mineral has specific roles to play. Here are some examples of the functions of micronutrients:

Vitamin A: Essential for vision, immune function, and cell growth and differentiation. It is found in foods like carrots, sweet potatoes, spinach, and liver.

Vitamin D: Important for calcium absorption and bone health. It can be synthesized by the body when the skin is exposed to sunlight, and it is also found in fatty fish, fortified dairy products, and egg yolks.

Vitamin E: Acts as an antioxidant, protecting cells from damage caused by free radicals. It is found in nuts, seeds, vegetable oils, and leafy green vegetables.

Vitamin K: Necessary for blood clotting and bone health. It is found in leafy green vegetables, broccoli, and vegetable oils.

B Vitamins: Play a crucial role in energy metabolism, nerve function, and red blood cell production. They are found in a variety of foods, including whole grains, legumes, meat, fish, and dairy products.

Vitamin C: Acts as an antioxidant, supports immune function, and aids in collagen synthesis. It is abundant in citrus fruits, strawberries, bell peppers, and broccoli.

Calcium: Essential for bone health, muscle function, and nerve transmission. It is found in dairy products, leafy green vegetables, and fortified foods.

Iron: Necessary for oxygen transport and energy production. It is found in red meat, poultry, fish, legumes, and fortified cereals.

Zinc: Important for immune function, wound healing, and DNA synthesis. It is found in meat, shellfish, legumes, and whole grains.

Iodine: Essential for thyroid hormone production, which regulates metabolism. It is found in iodized salt, seafood, and dairy products.

Meeting Micronutrient Needs through Diet

To ensure an adequate intake of micronutrients, it is important to consume a varied and balanced diet that includes a wide range of nutrient-dense foods. Here are some tips to help you meet your micronutrient needs:

Eat a variety of fruits and vegetables: Different fruits and vegetables contain different vitamins and minerals. Aim to include a colorful assortment of fruits and vegetables in your diet to ensure a diverse micronutrient intake.

Choose whole grains: Whole grains, such as brown rice, quinoa, and whole wheat bread, are rich in B vitamins and minerals like magnesium and selenium. Opt for whole grain options whenever possible.

Include lean protein sources: Protein-rich foods, such as lean meats, poultry, fish, eggs, legumes, and tofu, provide essential amino acids and minerals like iron and zinc.

Consume dairy or dairy alternatives: Dairy products, like milk, yogurt, and cheese, are excellent sources of calcium and vitamin D. If you follow a dairy-free diet, choose fortified plant-based alternatives.

Incorporate nuts and seeds: Nuts and seeds are packed with micronutrients, including vitamin E, magnesium, and zinc. Enjoy a handful of almonds, walnuts, chia seeds, or flaxseeds as a snack or add them to your meals.

Consider fortified foods: Fortified foods, such as fortified cereals, plant-based milks, and nutritional yeast, can be a convenient way to increase your intake of certain vitamins and minerals.

Cook foods properly: Some vitamins and minerals are sensitive to heat and can be lost during cooking. To preserve the micronutrient content of your food, opt for cooking methods like steaming, stir-frying, or microwaving, which require shorter cooking times.

Avoid excessive processing: Highly processed foods often have reduced micronutrient content due to refining and manufacturing processes. Opt for whole, minimally processed foods whenever possible.

Consult a healthcare professional: If you have specific dietary restrictions, allergies, or medical conditions, it is advisable to consult a healthcare professional or registered dietitian to ensure you are meeting your micronutrient needs.

Remember, while supplements can be useful in certain situations, it is generally best to obtain micronutrients from whole foods as part of a balanced diet. By focusing on a variety of nutrient-dense foods, you can ensure that you are meeting your micronutrient needs and supporting your overall health and well-being.

Meeting Micronutrient Needs through Diet

Micronutrients are essential nutrients that our bodies need in small amounts to function properly. They include vitamins and minerals, which play crucial roles in various bodily processes such as metabolism, immune function, and cell growth. While macronutrients like carbohydrates, proteins, and fats provide energy, micronutrients are responsible for supporting overall health and preventing nutrient deficiencies.

Meeting your micronutrient needs through a balanced diet is essential for maintaining optimal health. Here are some key micronutrients and their food sources that you should include in your diet:

8.5.1 Vitamin A

Vitamin A is important for maintaining healthy vision, supporting immune function, and promoting cell growth. It can be found in foods such as carrots, sweet potatoes, spinach, kale, and liver. Including these foods in your diet can help ensure you meet your vitamin A needs.

8.5.2 Vitamin C

Vitamin C is a powerful antioxidant that supports immune function, collagen production, and iron absorption. Citrus fruits like oranges and grapefruits, strawberries, bell peppers, and broccoli are excellent sources of vitamin C. Including these foods in your diet can help boost your vitamin C intake.

8.5.3 Vitamin D

Vitamin D plays a crucial role in bone health, immune function, and calcium absorption. While our bodies can produce vitamin D when exposed to sunlight, it can also be obtained from dietary sources such as fatty fish (salmon, mackerel), fortified dairy products, and egg yolks. If you have limited sun exposure, it may be necessary to consider vitamin D supplements.

8.5.4 Calcium

Calcium is essential for strong bones and teeth, muscle function, and nerve transmission. Dairy products like milk, cheese, and yogurt are excellent sources of calcium. If you follow a plant-based diet, you can obtain calcium from fortified plant-based milk alternatives, tofu, leafy greens (kale, broccoli), and almonds.

8.5.5 Iron

Iron is necessary for the production of red blood cells and oxygen transport throughout the body. Good sources of iron include lean meats, poultry, fish, legumes (beans, lentils), tofu, spinach, and fortified cereals. Pairing iron-rich foods with vitamin C-rich foods can enhance iron absorption.

8.5.6 B Vitamins

B vitamins, including thiamin, riboflavin, niacin, vitamin B6, folate, and vitamin B12, are essential for energy production, brain function, and red blood cell formation. Whole grains, legumes, nuts, seeds, lean meats, poultry, fish, eggs, and leafy greens are all good sources of B vitamins. For vitamin B12, which is primarily found in animal products, individuals following a vegan diet may need to consider supplementation.

8.5.7 Zinc

Zinc is important for immune function, wound healing, and DNA synthesis. It can be found in foods such as oysters, beef, poultry, beans, nuts, and whole grains. Including these foods in your diet can help ensure you meet your zinc needs.

8.5.8 Magnesium

Magnesium is involved in over 300 biochemical reactions in the body, including energy production, muscle function, and bone health. Good sources of magnesium include leafy greens, nuts, seeds, whole grains, legumes, and dark chocolate.

8.5.9 Potassium

Potassium is essential for maintaining fluid balance, nerve function, and muscle contractions. Bananas, oranges, avocados, potatoes, spinach, and beans are all excellent sources of potassium.

Including these foods in your diet can help ensure you meet your potassium needs.

8.5.10 Iodine

Iodine is necessary for the production of thyroid hormones, which regulate metabolism and growth. Seafood, seaweed, iodized salt, and dairy products are good sources of iodine. However, it's important to consume iodized salt in moderation and be mindful of your overall sodium intake.

8.5.11 Selenium

Selenium is an antioxidant that supports thyroid function and helps protect against oxidative stress. Brazil nuts, seafood, poultry, eggs, and whole grains are all good sources of selenium. However, it's important not to consume excessive amounts of selenium, as it can be toxic in high doses.

8.5.12 Copper

Copper is involved in the production of red blood cells, collagen synthesis, and iron absorption. Shellfish, organ meats, nuts, seeds, whole grains, and legumes are all good sources of copper.

8.5.13 Manganese

Manganese is important for bone health, metabolism, and antioxidant function. Whole grains, nuts, seeds, legumes, and leafy greens are all good sources of manganese.

8.5.14 Chromium

Chromium is involved in glucose metabolism and may help regulate blood sugar levels. Broccoli, whole grains, nuts, and lean meats are good sources of chromium.

Including a variety of nutrient-dense foods in your diet can help ensure you meet your micronutrient needs. Aim to consume a wide range of fruits, vegetables, whole grains, lean proteins, and healthy fats to provide your body with the necessary vitamins and minerals it needs to function optimally. If you have specific dietary restrictions or concerns, consult with a registered dietitian or healthcare professional to ensure you are meeting your micronutrient needs through diet.

MEAL PLANNING

Benefits of Meal Planning

Meal planning is a crucial aspect of maintaining a balanced diet. It involves taking the time to carefully plan and prepare your meals in advance, ensuring that you have nutritious and well-balanced options readily available. While it may require some initial effort and organization, the benefits of meal planning are numerous and can greatly contribute to your overall health and well-being.

1. Promotes Healthy Eating Habits

One of the primary benefits of meal planning is that it promotes healthy eating habits. When you plan your meals in advance, you have the opportunity to incorporate a variety of nutrient-dense foods into your diet. By consciously selecting a range of fruits, vegetables, whole grains, lean proteins, and healthy fats, you can ensure that your meals are well-balanced and provide your body with the essential nutrients it needs.

Meal planning also allows you to control portion sizes and avoid excessive calorie intake. By pre-determining the quantities of each food item, you can prevent overeating and maintain a healthy weight. Additionally, when you have a plan in place, you are less likely to rely on unhealthy convenience foods or make impulsive choices that may not align with your dietary goals.

2. Saves Time and Money

Another significant advantage of meal planning is that it saves both time and money. By dedicating a specific time to plan your meals for the week, you can streamline your grocery shopping and cooking processes. This eliminates the need for frequent trips to the store and reduces the likelihood of impulse purchases. With a well-thought-out meal plan, you can make a comprehensive shopping list and buy only the necessary ingredients, minimizing food waste and saving money in the process.

Meal planning also saves time during the week. By preparing meals in advance, you can significantly reduce the amount of time spent in the kitchen on a daily basis. Whether it's prepping ingredients, cooking in bulk, or assembling ready-to-eat meals, having a plan allows you to efficiently manage your time and ensures that you always have a healthy meal option available, even on busy days.

3. Reduces Stress and Decision Fatigue

The act of meal planning can help alleviate stress and decision fatigue associated with daily meal choices. When you have a plan in place, you eliminate the need to constantly think about what to cook or eat. This can be particularly beneficial for individuals with busy schedules or those who struggle with making healthy choices spontaneously.

By having a predetermined meal plan, you can approach each day with a clear idea of what you will be eating, eliminating the stress of last-minute decisions. This can also help you resist the temptation of unhealthy food options or takeout when you're tired or pressed for time. With meal planning, you can confidently stick to your dietary goals and maintain a consistent and balanced eating routine.

4. Supports Weight Management Goals

Meal planning is an effective tool for individuals looking to manage their weight. By carefully selecting and portioning your meals in advance, you can control your calorie intake and ensure that you are consuming the appropriate amount of nutrients for your body's needs. This can be particularly helpful for individuals who are trying to lose weight or maintain a healthy weight.

When you have a meal plan, you are less likely to succumb to unhealthy food choices or indulge in excessive snacking. By having nutritious meals readily available, you can avoid impulsive decisions that may hinder your weight management goals. Additionally, meal planning allows you to incorporate a variety of foods into your diet, making it easier to adhere to a balanced and sustainable eating plan.

5. Enhances Nutritional Variety and Diversity

Meal planning encourages the incorporation of a wide range of foods into your diet, promoting nutritional variety and diversity. By intentionally selecting different fruits, vegetables, whole grains, proteins, and fats, you can ensure that your body receives a broad spectrum of essential vitamins, minerals, and antioxidants.

When you plan your meals in advance, you have the opportunity to experiment with new recipes and ingredients. This can help expand your culinary horizons and introduce you to a wider range of flavors and textures. By incorporating a diverse array of foods into your meal plan, you can prevent dietary monotony and ensure that you are meeting your nutritional needs.

In conclusion, meal planning offers numerous benefits for individuals seeking to maintain a balanced diet. From promoting healthy eating habits and saving time and money to reducing stress and supporting weight management goals, the advantages of meal planning are undeniable. By taking the time to plan and prepare your meals in advance, you can set yourself up for success and make significant strides towards achieving optimal health and well-being.

Steps to Effective Meal Planning

Meal planning is a crucial aspect of maintaining a balanced diet. It helps you stay organized, save time and money, and ensures that you have nutritious meals readily available. By taking the time to plan your meals in advance, you can make healthier choices, avoid impulsive food purchases, and reduce food waste. Here are some steps to help you create an effective meal plan:

Step 1: Set Your Goals and Consider Your Needs

Before you start meal planning, it's important to identify your goals and consider your specific dietary needs. Are you looking to lose weight, gain muscle, or simply maintain a healthy lifestyle? Do you have any dietary restrictions or allergies? Understanding your goals and needs will help you tailor your meal plan accordingly.

For example, if your goal is to lose weight, you may want to focus on creating a calorie deficit by incorporating more low-calorie, nutrient-dense foods into your meals. On the other hand, if you're an athlete looking to build muscle, you might need to increase your protein intake and include more complex carbohydrates in your meals.

Step 2: Create a Weekly Meal Schedule

Start by creating a weekly meal schedule that outlines what you'll be eating for each meal and snack throughout the week. Consider your schedule and plan meals that are convenient and easy to prepare on busy days. It's also helpful to designate specific days for meal prepping and batch cooking, which we'll discuss in more detail in the next section.

For example, you might plan to have a vegetable stir-fry with tofu and brown rice on Monday, a grilled chicken salad on Tuesday, a lentil curry with quinoa on Wednesday, and so on. Having a schedule in place will make grocery shopping and meal preparation much more efficient.

Step 3: Choose Nutrient-Dense Foods

When selecting foods for your meal plan, focus on nutrient-dense options that provide a wide range of vitamins, minerals, and antioxidants. Include a variety of fruits, vegetables, whole grains, lean proteins, and healthy fats in your meals.

For example, instead of opting for processed snacks, choose fresh fruits, nuts, or yogurt as healthier alternatives. Instead of white bread, choose whole grain bread for sandwiches. By making these small changes, you can significantly improve the nutritional value of your meals.

Step 4: Make a Grocery List

Once you have your meal schedule in place, create a grocery list based on the ingredients you'll need for each meal. Take inventory of your pantry and fridge to see what items you already have and what needs to be replenished. Organize your list by food groups or sections of the grocery store to make shopping more efficient.

For example, if you're planning to make a vegetable stir-fry, your grocery list might include ingredients like broccoli, bell peppers, carrots, tofu, and brown rice. By having a well-organized grocery list, you'll be less likely to forget any essential items and avoid unnecessary trips to the store.

Step 5: Shop and Prep

With your grocery list in hand, head to the store and purchase the items you need. Try to stick to your list and avoid impulse purchases that may derail your meal plan. Once you're back home, take some time to wash, chop, and prep your ingredients.

For example, you can wash and chop your vegetables, cook grains and proteins in advance, and portion out snacks for the week. This will make it easier and quicker to assemble your meals during the week, especially on busy days when you may not have much time to cook.

Step 6: Cook and Store

As you progress through the week, follow your meal schedule and prepare your meals according to your plan. Cook in batches whenever possible, so you have leftovers that can be enjoyed for future meals. Invest in quality food storage containers to keep your meals fresh and easily accessible.

For example, if you're making a large pot of soup, divide it into individual portions and store them in the freezer for later use. This way, you'll always have a healthy meal option available, even on days when you don't feel like cooking.

Step 7: Evaluate and Adjust

After a week or two of following your meal plan, take some time to evaluate how it's working for you. Are you enjoying the meals? Are you meeting your nutritional goals? Are there any adjustments you need to make?

For example, if you find that you're not enjoying a particular meal or it's not keeping you satisfied, consider making changes to the recipe or replacing it with a different option. Meal planning is a flexible process, and it's important to adapt it to your preferences and needs.

By following these steps, you can create an effective meal plan that supports your health and wellness goals. Remember, meal planning is a skill that takes practice, so don't be discouraged if it takes some time to find a routine that works best for you. With consistency and dedication, you'll soon reap the benefits of a well-planned and balanced diet.

Meal Prepping and Batch Cooking

Meal prepping and batch cooking are two strategies that can greatly simplify the process of eating a balanced diet. These techniques involve preparing and cooking larger quantities of food in advance, which can save time, money, and effort throughout the week. By dedicating a few hours to meal prepping and batch cooking, you can ensure that you have nutritious meals readily available, even on your busiest days.

Benefits of Meal Prepping and Batch Cooking

There are numerous benefits to incorporating meal prepping and batch cooking into your routine. Here are some of the key advantages:

Time-saving: By dedicating a few hours on a specific day to prepare meals for the week, you can save a significant amount of time during the rest of the week. Instead of spending time each day planning and cooking meals, you can simply reheat the pre-prepared meals and enjoy a nutritious and balanced diet without the hassle.

Cost-effective: Meal prepping and batch cooking can also help you save money. By buying ingredients in bulk and utilizing them efficiently, you can reduce food waste and make the most of your grocery budget. Additionally, by having meals ready to go, you are less likely to rely on expensive takeout or convenience foods.

Portion control: When you prepare meals in advance, you have more control over portion sizes. This can be particularly beneficial if you are trying to manage your weight or adhere to specific dietary guidelines. By portioning out your meals in advance, you can ensure that you are consuming appropriate amounts of each food group.

Nutritional balance: Meal prepping and batch cooking allow you to plan and prepare meals that are nutritionally balanced. You can ensure that each meal includes a variety of macronutrients (carbohydrates, proteins, and fats) as well as a range of micronutrients (vitamins and minerals). This can help support overall health and well-being.

Tips for Meal Prepping and Batch Cooking

To make the most of meal prepping and batch cooking, consider the following tips:

Plan your meals: Before you start cooking, take some time to plan your meals for the week. Consider your dietary needs, preferences, and any specific goals you may have. This will help you create a shopping list and ensure that you have all the necessary ingredients on hand.

Choose versatile ingredients: Opt for ingredients that can be used in multiple dishes. For example, roasted vegetables can be added to salads, grain bowls, or wraps. This will help you create a variety of meals using the same base ingredients.

Invest in quality storage containers: To keep your pre-prepared meals fresh and safe to eat, invest in high-quality storage containers. Look for containers that are microwave-safe, leak-proof, and stackable for easy storage in the refrigerator or freezer.

Label and date your meals: To avoid confusion and ensure that you consume meals before they spoil, label and date each container. This will help you keep track of how long each meal has been stored and prioritize meals that need to be consumed first.

Consider freezing meals: If you are batch cooking and have prepared more meals than you can consume within a few days, consider freezing some portions. Freezing meals can extend their shelf life and provide you with a variety of options to choose from in the future.

Mix and match: Don't be afraid to mix and match ingredients to create new and exciting meals. For example, you can use pre-cooked chicken in salads, wraps, or stir-fries. This will help prevent meal fatigue and keep your taste buds satisfied.

Stay organized: Keep your kitchen organized and clean while meal prepping and batch cooking. This will make the process more efficient and enjoyable. Clean as you go, and make sure to store ingredients properly to maintain their freshness.

Meal Prepping for Different Dietary Needs

Meal prepping and batch cooking can be adapted to suit various dietary needs and preferences. Here are some examples:

Vegetarian or vegan meal prepping: If you follow a vegetarian or vegan diet, you can focus on incorporating plant-based proteins such as legumes, tofu, tempeh, or seitan into your meals. Prepare a variety of vegetable-based dishes, grain bowls, and salads to ensure a balanced and satisfying diet.

Gluten-free meal prepping: For individuals with gluten intolerance or celiac disease, it's important to choose gluten-free grains such as quinoa, rice, or gluten-free oats. Incorporate a variety of vegetables, lean proteins, and healthy fats to create well-rounded gluten-free meals.

Low-carb or keto meal prepping: If you are following a low-carb or ketogenic diet, focus on incorporating non-starchy vegetables, healthy fats, and moderate amounts of protein into your meals. Prepare dishes such as roasted vegetables, grilled chicken or fish, and avocado-based salads.

Allergen-free meal prepping: If you have food allergies or intolerances, it's crucial to avoid the specific allergens. Plan meals that exclude the allergenic ingredients and focus on incorporating safe alternatives. For example, if you have a dairy allergy, use plant-based milk and dairy-free cheese substitutes.

Remember, it's always a good idea to consult with a healthcare professional or registered dietitian before making significant changes to your diet, especially if you have specific dietary needs or medical conditions.

By incorporating meal prepping and batch cooking into your routine, you can simplify the process of eating a balanced diet. These strategies can help you save time, money, and effort while ensuring that you have nutritious meals readily available. Experiment with different recipes, ingredients, and flavors to keep your meals exciting and enjoyable.

Meal Planning for Different Dietary Needs

Meal planning is a valuable tool for individuals looking to maintain a balanced diet. It allows you to carefully consider your nutritional needs and preferences while ensuring that you have a variety of healthy and delicious meals throughout the week. While meal planning is beneficial for everyone, it becomes even more important when considering different dietary needs. In this section, we will explore meal planning strategies for various dietary requirements, including vegetarian, vegan, gluten-free, and dairy-free diets.

Vegetarian Meal Planning

Vegetarianism is a dietary choice that excludes meat, poultry, and seafood. However, it still allows for the consumption of plant-based foods such as fruits, vegetables, grains, legumes, nuts, and seeds. When meal planning for vegetarians, it is essential to ensure that meals are nutritionally balanced and provide adequate protein, iron, calcium, and vitamin B12.

Here are some meal planning tips for vegetarians:

Incorporate a variety of plant-based protein sources such as tofu, tempeh, legumes, and quinoa into your meals.

Include iron-rich foods like leafy greens, lentils, and fortified cereals to meet your iron needs.

Ensure sufficient calcium intake by including dairy alternatives like fortified plant-based milk, tofu, and leafy greens.

Consider incorporating vitamin B12-fortified foods or supplements to meet your B12 requirements.

Vegan Meal Planning

Veganism takes vegetarianism a step further by excluding all animal products, including dairy, eggs, and honey. When meal planning for vegans, it is crucial to ensure that meals are nutritionally balanced and provide adequate protein, iron, calcium, vitamin B12, and omega-3 fatty acids.

Here are some meal planning tips for vegans:

Include a variety of plant-based protein sources such as legumes, tofu, tempeh, seitan, and quinoa.

Incorporate iron-rich foods like leafy greens, lentils, beans, and fortified cereals into your meals.

Ensure sufficient calcium intake by including fortified plant-based milk, tofu, leafy greens, and calcium-fortified foods.

Consider incorporating vitamin B12-fortified foods or supplements to meet your B12 requirements.

Include plant-based sources of omega-3 fatty acids, such as flaxseeds, chia seeds, hemp seeds, and walnuts.

Gluten-Free Meal Planning

A gluten-free diet is essential for individuals with celiac disease or gluten sensitivity. Gluten is a protein found in wheat, barley, and rye. When meal planning for a gluten-free diet, it is crucial to avoid all sources of gluten and ensure that meals are nutritionally balanced and provide adequate fiber, vitamins, and minerals.

Here are some meal planning tips for a gluten-free diet:

Choose naturally gluten-free grains like rice, quinoa, millet, and corn as the base for your meals.

Incorporate a variety of fruits and vegetables to ensure a wide range of vitamins and minerals.

Include gluten-free sources of fiber such as beans, lentils, nuts, and seeds.

Read food labels carefully to avoid hidden sources of gluten in processed foods.

Consider gluten-free alternatives for bread, pasta, and other grain-based products.

Dairy-Free Meal Planning

A dairy-free diet excludes all dairy products, including milk, cheese, yogurt, and butter. This dietary choice is often made by individuals with lactose intolerance or dairy allergies. When meal planning for a dairy-free diet, it is important to ensure that meals are nutritionally balanced and provide adequate calcium, vitamin D, and other essential nutrients typically found in dairy products.

Here are some meal planning tips for a dairy-free diet:

Choose calcium-fortified plant-based milk alternatives like almond milk, soy milk, or oat milk.

Include calcium-rich foods such as leafy greens, tofu, fortified cereals, and canned fish with bones.

Consider incorporating other sources of vitamin D, such as fortified plant-based milk or spending time in the sun.

Experiment with dairy-free alternatives for cheese, yogurt, and butter, such as nut-based cheeses or coconut-based yogurt.

Remember, it is always a good idea to consult with a registered dietitian or healthcare professional when making significant dietary changes or if you have specific dietary needs. They can provide personalized guidance and ensure that your meal plan meets your nutritional requirements.

By considering different dietary needs in your meal planning, you can create a diverse and satisfying menu that caters to a range of preferences and requirements. Whether you follow a vegetarian, vegan, gluten-free, or dairy-free diet, meal planning allows you to enjoy delicious and nutritious meals while maintaining a balanced diet.

DIETARY GUIDELINES

Understanding Dietary Guidelines

Dietary guidelines are a set of recommendations provided by health organizations and government agencies to promote optimal nutrition and overall health. These guidelines are based on scientific research and aim to provide individuals with the necessary information to make informed decisions about their food choices. Understanding dietary guidelines is essential for maintaining a balanced diet and achieving optimal health.

Dietary guidelines typically include recommendations for various food groups, portion sizes, nutrient intake, and overall dietary patterns. They are designed to address the specific nutritional needs of different populations and age groups. By following these guidelines, individuals can ensure that they are consuming a variety of nutrients and maintaining a healthy balance of macronutrients and micronutrients.

The specific recommendations provided in dietary guidelines may vary depending on the country or organization that issues them. However, they generally emphasize the importance of consuming a variety of nutrient-dense foods while limiting the intake of unhealthy fats, added sugars, and sodium. Let's take a closer look at some national and international dietary guidelines to understand their key principles.

National and International Dietary Guidelines

United States Dietary Guidelines for Americans

The United States Dietary Guidelines for Americans are updated every five years by the U.S. Department of Agriculture (USDA) and the Department of Health and Human Services (HHS). These guidelines provide evidence-based recommendations for Americans aged two years and older to promote health, prevent chronic diseases, and maintain a healthy weight.

The key principles of the U.S. Dietary Guidelines for Americans include:

Balancing Calories: The guidelines emphasize the importance of balancing calorie intake with physical activity to maintain a healthy weight. They recommend consuming nutrient-dense foods while limiting the intake of added sugars, saturated fats, and sodium.

Food Groups to Encourage: The guidelines encourage individuals to consume a variety of fruits, vegetables, whole grains, lean proteins, and low-fat dairy products. These food groups provide essential nutrients and contribute to a balanced diet.

Reducing Sodium, Added Sugars, and Saturated Fats: The guidelines recommend reducing the intake of sodium, added sugars, and saturated fats. This can be achieved by choosing foods with lower sodium content, limiting the consumption of sugary beverages and snacks, and opting for lean sources of protein.

Shift to Healthier Food and Beverage Choices: The guidelines encourage individuals to make healthier food and beverage choices. This includes replacing sugary drinks with water, choosing whole grains over refined grains, and opting for lean sources of protein.

World Health Organization (WHO) Dietary Guidelines

The World Health Organization (WHO) provides dietary guidelines that are applicable globally. These guidelines aim to promote health, prevent chronic diseases, and reduce the risk of malnutrition.

The key principles of the WHO Dietary Guidelines include:

Balanced Diet: The guidelines emphasize the importance of consuming a balanced diet that includes a variety of fruits, vegetables, whole grains, legumes, nuts, and seeds. This ensures the intake of essential nutrients and promotes overall health.

Limiting the Intake of Unhealthy Fats and Sugars: The guidelines recommend limiting the consumption of unhealthy fats, such as saturated and trans fats, and reducing the intake of added sugars. This can be achieved by choosing healthier cooking oils, avoiding processed foods high in unhealthy fats, and reducing the consumption of sugary snacks and beverages.

Promoting Physical Activity: The guidelines highlight the importance of regular physical activity for maintaining a healthy weight and overall well-being. They recommend engaging in at least 150 minutes of moderate-intensity aerobic activity or 75 minutes of vigorous-intensity aerobic activity per week.

Promoting Breastfeeding: The guidelines emphasize the importance of exclusive breastfeeding for the first six months of life and continued breastfeeding along with appropriate complementary foods up to two years of age or beyond. Breastfeeding provides essential nutrients and promotes optimal growth and development in infants.

Applying Dietary Guidelines to Your Diet

To apply dietary guidelines to your diet, it is important to understand your individual nutritional needs and make appropriate adjustments. Here are some tips for incorporating dietary guidelines into your daily routine:

Eat a Variety of Nutrient-Dense Foods: Include a wide range of fruits, vegetables, whole grains, lean proteins, and healthy fats in your meals. This ensures that you are getting a diverse array of essential nutrients.

Limit Added Sugars and Unhealthy Fats: Be mindful of the amount of added sugars and unhealthy fats in your diet. Read food labels and choose products with lower sugar and fat content. Opt for cooking methods that use less oil and avoid deep-fried foods.

Control Portion Sizes: Pay attention to portion sizes to avoid overeating. Use smaller plates and bowls, and listen to your body's hunger and fullness cues. Avoid eating large portions of high-calorie foods.

Stay Hydrated: Drink an adequate amount of water throughout the day to maintain proper hydration. Limit the consumption of sugary beverages and opt for water, herbal tea, or infused water instead.

Be Mindful of Sodium Intake: Limit the consumption of high-sodium foods, such as processed meats, canned soups, and salty snacks. Opt for fresh or homemade meals that allow you to control the amount of salt added.

Engage in Regular Physical Activity: Incorporate regular physical activity into your routine to support overall health and weight management. Aim for a combination of cardiovascular exercise, strength training, and flexibility exercises.

By following these guidelines and making conscious choices about your food intake, you can ensure that you are nourishing your body with the nutrients it needs for optimal health. Remember that dietary guidelines are meant to be flexible and adaptable to individual needs, so feel free to make adjustments based on your specific circumstances and preferences.

National and International Dietary Guidelines

National and international dietary guidelines play a crucial role in promoting and maintaining a balanced diet for individuals and populations. These guidelines are developed by various organizations and governmental bodies to provide evidence-based recommendations on healthy eating patterns and food choices. By following these guidelines, individuals can make informed decisions about their diet and improve their overall health and well-being.

Importance of National and International Dietary Guidelines

National and international dietary guidelines serve as a framework for individuals, healthcare professionals, policymakers, and food industries to understand the nutritional needs of the population and develop strategies to address public health concerns. These guidelines are based on extensive research and scientific evidence, taking into account various factors such as age, sex, activity level, and specific health conditions.

The primary objectives of these guidelines are to:

Promote health and prevent chronic diseases: National and international dietary guidelines aim to reduce the risk of chronic diseases such as obesity, diabetes, cardiovascular diseases, and certain types of cancer. By providing recommendations on nutrient intake and food choices, these guidelines help individuals adopt healthier eating habits and reduce their risk of developing these conditions.

Ensure nutrient adequacy: Dietary guidelines emphasize the importance of consuming a variety of nutrient-dense foods to meet the body's nutritional needs. They provide guidance on the recommended intake of macronutrients (carbohydrates, proteins, and fats) and micronutrients (vitamins and minerals) to support optimal health and prevent nutrient deficiencies.

Promote sustainability: Many national and international dietary guidelines now include recommendations on sustainable eating practices. These guidelines encourage individuals to choose foods that have a lower environmental impact, such as plant-based options, and reduce food waste. By promoting sustainable eating, these guidelines aim to protect the environment and ensure the availability of nutritious food for future generations.

Examples of National and International Dietary Guidelines

Different countries and organizations have developed their own national and international dietary guidelines to address the specific needs and cultural preferences of their populations. Here are a few examples:

United States Dietary Guidelines for Americans: The U.S. Department of Agriculture (USDA) and the Department of Health and Human Services (HHS) jointly publish the Dietary Guidelines for Americans every five years. These guidelines provide evidence-based recommendations on healthy eating patterns, nutrient intake, and physical activity. They emphasize the consumption of fruits, vegetables, whole grains, lean proteins, and low-fat dairy products while limiting added sugars, saturated fats, and sodium.

European Food Safety Authority (EFSA) Dietary Reference Values: EFSA provides scientific advice on nutrient intake for the European Union (EU) member states. Their dietary reference values include recommended daily intakes of macronutrients, vitamins, and minerals for different age groups and population subgroups. These guidelines help ensure that individuals in Europe meet their nutritional needs and maintain good health.

Australian Dietary Guidelines: The Australian Dietary Guidelines are developed by the National Health and Medical Research Council (NHMRC) and provide recommendations on healthy eating patterns to promote health and prevent chronic diseases. These guidelines emphasize the consumption of a variety of fruits, vegetables, whole grains, lean proteins, and dairy products while limiting added sugars, salt, and saturated fats.

World Health Organization (WHO) Global Dietary Guidelines: The WHO provides global dietary guidelines that aim to promote healthy eating patterns and prevent non-communicable diseases. These guidelines emphasize the consumption of a balanced diet that includes a variety of fruits, vegetables, whole grains, legumes, nuts, and seeds while limiting the intake of processed foods, sugary beverages, and unhealthy fats.

Applying National and International Dietary Guidelines to Your Diet

To apply national and international dietary guidelines to your diet, consider the following tips:

Familiarize yourself with the guidelines: Take the time to read and understand the specific recommendations provided in the national or international dietary guidelines relevant to your country or region. Pay attention to the recommended food groups, portion sizes, and nutrient intake.

Plan your meals: Use the dietary guidelines as a basis for planning your meals. Aim to include a variety of foods from different food groups to ensure a balanced intake of macronutrients and micronutrients. Consider incorporating fruits, vegetables, whole grains, lean proteins, and healthy fats into your meals.

Make gradual changes: If your current diet does not align with the dietary guidelines, start by making small, sustainable changes. For example, gradually increase your intake of fruits and vegetables, choose whole grains over refined grains, and opt for lean sources of protein.

Seek professional advice: If you have specific dietary needs or health conditions, consult a registered dietitian or healthcare professional who can provide personalized guidance based on the national or international dietary guidelines. They can help you develop a meal plan that meets your nutritional requirements and supports your health goals.

Remember, national and international dietary guidelines are meant to serve as a general framework for healthy eating. It's important to adapt these guidelines to your individual needs, preferences, and cultural considerations. By incorporating the principles of balanced nutrition outlined in the guidelines, you can make informed choices that support your overall health and well-being.

Applying Dietary Guidelines to Your Diet

Once you have a good understanding of dietary guidelines and their importance, the next step is to apply them to your own diet. This section will provide you with practical tips and strategies to incorporate these guidelines into your daily eating habits. By following these recommendations, you can ensure that you are nourishing your body with the right nutrients and maintaining a balanced diet.

Start with a Solid Foundation

The foundation of a balanced diet lies in consuming a variety of nutrient-dense foods from all the food groups. This means including fruits, vegetables, whole grains, lean proteins, and healthy fats in your meals. Aim to fill half of your plate with fruits and vegetables, one-quarter with whole grains, and one-quarter with lean proteins. This balanced approach ensures that you are getting a wide range of essential nutrients.

For example, you can start your day with a bowl of oatmeal topped with fresh berries and a sprinkle of nuts. This breakfast provides a good balance of carbohydrates, fiber, protein, and healthy fats. For lunch, you can have a salad with mixed greens, grilled chicken, avocado, and a drizzle of olive oil. This meal incorporates vegetables, lean protein, and healthy fats. For dinner, you can enjoy a stir-fry with a variety of colorful vegetables, tofu or shrimp, and brown rice. This dish includes a mix of vegetables, protein, and whole grains.

Be Mindful of Portion Sizes

While it's important to include a variety of foods in your diet, it's equally important to be mindful of portion sizes. Even healthy foods can contribute to weight gain if consumed in excessive amounts. Use the portion control tips discussed in Chapter 4 to help you manage your serving sizes.

For instance, when enjoying a pasta dish, measure out a serving size of cooked pasta (about half a cup) and fill the rest of your plate with vegetables and lean protein. This way, you can still enjoy your favorite foods while keeping your portions in check. Remember, it's not about depriving yourself, but rather finding a balance that works for you.

Limit Added Sugars and Sodium

Dietary guidelines often emphasize the importance of limiting added sugars and sodium in your diet. Added sugars can contribute to weight gain and increase the risk of chronic diseases, while excessive sodium intake can lead to high blood pressure and other health issues.

To reduce your intake of added sugars, opt for whole fruits instead of sugary snacks or desserts. Choose unsweetened beverages like water, herbal tea, or infused water instead of sugary drinks.

When it comes to sodium, read food labels carefully and choose low-sodium options whenever possible. Flavor your meals with herbs, spices, and other seasonings instead of relying on salt.

Make Smart Substitutions

Another way to apply dietary guidelines to your diet is by making smart substitutions. For example, instead of using refined grains like white bread or white rice, opt for whole grain alternatives like whole wheat bread or brown rice. These options provide more fiber and nutrients.

When it comes to fats, choose healthy sources like avocados, nuts, and olive oil instead of saturated and trans fats found in fried foods and processed snacks. These healthier fats can help support heart health and provide essential nutrients.

Plan and Prepare Meals in Advance

Meal planning and preparation can greatly assist in applying dietary guidelines to your diet. By planning your meals in advance, you can ensure that you have a variety of nutritious options available and avoid relying on unhealthy convenience foods.

Take some time each week to plan your meals, create a shopping list, and prepare ingredients in advance. This way, you can make healthier choices and have meals ready to go when you're busy or tired. Consider batch cooking and meal prepping to save time and ensure that you always have nutritious meals on hand.

Seek Professional Guidance

If you find it challenging to apply dietary guidelines to your diet or have specific dietary needs, it may be helpful to seek guidance from a registered dietitian or nutritionist. These professionals can provide personalized recommendations based on your individual needs and goals.

They can help you create a meal plan that aligns with dietary guidelines and address any concerns or questions you may have. Working with a professional can provide you with the support and knowledge you need to make sustainable changes to your diet.

Remember, applying dietary guidelines to your diet is a journey, and it's important to be patient with yourself. Start by making small changes and gradually incorporate healthier habits into your routine. Over time, these changes will become second nature, and you will reap the benefits of a balanced diet and improved overall health.

Evaluating and Adapting Dietary Guidelines

Dietary guidelines are an essential tool for promoting and maintaining a balanced diet. They provide recommendations on the types and amounts of food that individuals should consume to meet their nutritional needs and support overall health. However, it is important to understand that dietary guidelines are not one-size-fits-all. Each person has unique dietary requirements based on factors such as age, sex, activity level, and underlying health conditions. Therefore, it is crucial to evaluate and adapt dietary guidelines to suit individual needs.

Evaluating Dietary Guidelines

When evaluating dietary guidelines, it is important to consider the source and the scientific evidence behind the recommendations. National and international organizations, such as the United States Department of Agriculture (USDA) and the World Health Organization (WHO), develop dietary guidelines based on extensive research and expert consensus. These guidelines are regularly updated to reflect the latest scientific findings.

To evaluate dietary guidelines, consider the following factors:

Scientific Basis: Look for guidelines that are based on a robust body of scientific evidence. Guidelines that are supported by multiple studies and research findings are more likely to be reliable and accurate.

Transparency: Ensure that the guidelines provide clear information about the methodology used to develop the recommendations. Look for guidelines that are transparent about the sources of evidence and the process of reviewing and updating the guidelines.

Consistency: Check if the guidelines align with other reputable sources of nutrition information. Consistency among different organizations and experts adds credibility to the guidelines.

Applicability: Consider whether the guidelines are applicable to your specific demographic group or health condition. Some guidelines may be tailored to specific populations, such as children, pregnant women, or individuals with chronic diseases.

Practicality: Assess whether the guidelines are practical and feasible to implement in your daily life. Guidelines that are overly restrictive or difficult to follow may not be sustainable in the long term.

By critically evaluating dietary guidelines, you can make informed decisions about which recommendations to incorporate into your own balanced diet.

Adapting Dietary Guidelines

While dietary guidelines provide a valuable framework for healthy eating, they may need to be adapted to meet individual needs and preferences. Here are some considerations for adapting dietary guidelines:

Personalized Calorie Needs: The calorie recommendations in dietary guidelines are typically based on average requirements. However, individual calorie needs can vary based on factors such as age, sex, weight, and activity level. Consult with a healthcare professional or registered dietitian to determine your specific calorie needs.

Food Preferences and Allergies: Dietary guidelines often provide general recommendations for food groups and nutrient intake. However, it is important to adapt these recommendations to accommodate personal food preferences and any allergies or intolerances. For example, if you have a dairy allergy, you can substitute dairy products with alternative sources of calcium, such as fortified plant-based milks or leafy green vegetables.

Cultural and Ethnic Considerations: Dietary guidelines may not always reflect the diverse food traditions and cultural practices of different populations. It is important to adapt the guidelines to incorporate culturally appropriate foods and cooking methods. For example, if a dietary guideline recommends consuming whole grains, you can choose traditional whole grain options that are commonly consumed in your culture.

Individual Health Conditions: Individuals with specific health conditions, such as diabetes, heart disease, or gastrointestinal disorders, may need to modify dietary guidelines to manage their condition effectively. Consult with a healthcare professional or registered dietitian who specializes in your specific health condition for personalized dietary recommendations.

Lifestyle and Activity Level: Consider your lifestyle and activity level when adapting dietary guidelines. If you have a physically demanding job or engage in regular exercise, you may need to adjust your nutrient intake to support your energy needs and muscle recovery.

Remember, the goal is to create a balanced diet that meets your individual needs while adhering to the core principles of a healthy eating pattern. By evaluating and adapting dietary guidelines, you can create a personalized approach to nutrition that supports your overall health and well-being.

SPECIAL DIES FOR SPECIAL CLASSES OF PEOPLE

Balanced Diet for Children and Adolescents

Children and adolescents have unique nutritional needs due to their rapid growth and development. A balanced diet plays a crucial role in supporting their physical and cognitive growth, as well as maintaining their overall health and well-being. Providing them with the right nutrients in appropriate quantities is essential for their optimal growth and development.

Nutritional Needs of Children

Children require a well-balanced diet that includes a variety of nutrients to support their growth and development. Here are some key nutrients that are particularly important for children:

Protein: Protein is essential for the growth and repair of tissues, as well as the production of enzymes and hormones. Good sources of protein for children include lean meats, poultry, fish, eggs, dairy products, legumes, and nuts.

Carbohydrates: Carbohydrates are the primary source of energy for children. Complex carbohydrates, such as whole grains, fruits, vegetables, and legumes, provide essential vitamins, minerals, and fiber. These should be the main source of carbohydrates in a child's diet, while sugary snacks and beverages should be limited.

Fats: Healthy fats are important for brain development and the absorption of fat-soluble vitamins. Children should consume sources of healthy fats, such as avocados, nuts, seeds, olive oil, and fatty fish like salmon. Limiting saturated and trans fats found in processed foods is crucial for their overall health.

Calcium: Calcium is essential for the development of strong bones and teeth. Dairy products like milk, cheese, and yogurt are excellent sources of calcium. For children who are lactose intolerant or have dairy allergies, calcium can be obtained from fortified plant-based milk alternatives, tofu, leafy green vegetables, and fortified cereals.

Iron: Iron is necessary for the production of red blood cells and oxygen transport throughout the body. Good sources of iron include lean meats, poultry, fish, fortified cereals, beans, lentils, and leafy green vegetables. Iron absorption can be enhanced by consuming vitamin C-rich foods, such as citrus fruits, strawberries, and bell peppers, alongside iron-rich foods.

Vitamins and Minerals: Children require a wide range of vitamins and minerals for their overall growth and development. Encouraging them to consume a variety of fruits, vegetables, whole grains, lean proteins, and dairy products will help ensure they receive an adequate intake of essential vitamins and minerals.

Establishing Healthy Eating Habits

It is important to establish healthy eating habits in children from an early age. Here are some tips to promote a balanced diet for children and adolescents:

Lead by Example: Children are more likely to adopt healthy eating habits if they see their parents and caregivers practicing them. Be a role model by consuming a balanced diet and involving them in meal planning and preparation.

Offer a Variety of Foods: Introduce a wide range of foods to children, including fruits, vegetables, whole grains, lean proteins, and dairy products. Encourage them to try new foods and flavors, and involve them in grocery shopping and meal preparation to increase their interest in healthy eating.

Limit Processed Foods and Sugary Drinks: Minimize the consumption of processed foods, such as fast food, sugary snacks, and beverages. These foods are often high in unhealthy fats, added sugars, and sodium, which can negatively impact children's health.

Encourage Regular Meals and Snacks: Establish regular meal and snack times to ensure children receive adequate nutrition throughout the day. Offer a combination of protein, carbohydrates, and healthy fats in each meal to provide sustained energy and promote satiety.

Promote Hydration: Encourage children to drink water throughout the day to stay hydrated. Limit the consumption of sugary drinks, such as soda and fruit juices, as they can contribute to excessive calorie intake and dental issues.

Limit Screen Time: Excessive screen time can lead to sedentary behavior and unhealthy eating habits. Encourage children to engage in physical activities and limit their screen time to promote a healthy lifestyle.

Addressing Special Dietary Needs

Some children may have special dietary needs due to allergies, intolerances, or medical conditions. It is important to work closely with healthcare professionals, such as pediatricians and registered dietitians, to develop appropriate meal plans and ensure nutritional adequacy.

For children with allergies or intolerances, it is crucial to identify and eliminate the specific allergens or intolerant foods from their diet. This may require careful label reading and meal planning to avoid cross-contamination and ensure their nutritional needs are met.

Children with medical conditions, such as diabetes or celiac disease, may require specific dietary modifications. Working with healthcare professionals will help create individualized meal plans that meet their unique needs while still providing a balanced diet.

Conclusion

A balanced diet is essential for the growth, development, and overall health of children and adolescents. By providing them with a variety of nutrient-dense foods and establishing healthy eating habits from an early age, we can set them on a path towards a lifetime of good health. Remember to lead by example, offer a variety of foods, limit processed foods and sugary drinks, encourage regular meals and snacks, promote hydration, and address any special dietary needs.

Balanced Diet for Pregnant and Nursing Women

Pregnancy and breastfeeding are crucial periods in a woman's life that require special attention to nutrition. During these stages, the body undergoes significant changes, and the nutritional needs increase to support the growth and development of the baby. A balanced diet becomes even more important to ensure both the mother and the baby receive adequate nutrients. In this section, we will explore the specific dietary considerations for pregnant and nursing women and provide practical tips for maintaining a balanced diet.

Nutritional Needs during Pregnancy

Pregnancy is a time of increased nutrient requirements to support the growth and development of the fetus. It is essential for pregnant women to consume a variety of nutrient-dense foods to meet these increased needs. Here are some key nutrients that pregnant women should focus on:

Folic Acid: Adequate intake of folic acid is crucial during the early stages of pregnancy to prevent neural tube defects in the baby. Good sources of folic acid include leafy green vegetables, citrus fruits, legumes, and fortified grains.

Iron: Iron is necessary for the production of red blood cells and to prevent anemia. Pregnant women require more iron to support the increased blood volume and the development of the baby. Iron-rich foods include lean meats, poultry, fish, fortified cereals, and dark leafy greens.

Calcium: Calcium is essential for the development of the baby's bones and teeth. Pregnant women should aim to consume adequate amounts of dairy products, fortified plant-based milk, tofu, and leafy green vegetables.

Protein: Protein is crucial for the growth and development of the baby's tissues. Good sources of protein include lean meats, poultry, fish, eggs, dairy products, legumes, and nuts.

Omega-3 Fatty Acids: Omega-3 fatty acids, particularly DHA (docosahexaenoic acid), play a vital role in the development of the baby's brain and eyes. Good sources of omega-3 fatty acids include fatty fish (such as salmon and sardines), walnuts, flaxseeds, and chia seeds.

Meal Planning for Pregnant Women

To ensure a balanced diet during pregnancy, it is important to plan meals that incorporate a variety of nutrient-rich foods. Here is an example of a day's meal plan for a pregnant woman:

Breakfast: A bowl of fortified cereal with milk, topped with fresh berries and a handful of nuts.

Snack: Greek yogurt with sliced fruits.

Lunch: Grilled chicken breast with a side of steamed vegetables and quinoa.

Snack: Carrot sticks with hummus.

Dinner: Baked salmon with roasted sweet potatoes and a side salad.

Snack: A small handful of almonds.

Remember to include a variety of fruits, vegetables, whole grains, lean proteins, and healthy fats in your meals. It is also important to stay hydrated by drinking plenty of water throughout the day.

Nutritional Needs during Breastfeeding

Breastfeeding is a demanding process that requires additional energy and nutrients. The quality of breast milk is directly influenced by the mother's diet, so it is crucial to maintain a balanced diet to ensure optimal nutrition for both the mother and the baby. Here are some key nutrients to focus on during breastfeeding:

Calories: Breastfeeding women require additional calories to support milk production. It is recommended to consume an extra 500 calories per day, but individual needs may vary. Focus on nutrient-dense foods to meet these additional calorie needs.

Fluids: Staying hydrated is essential for milk production. Aim to drink plenty of water throughout the day. It is also beneficial to include other hydrating beverages such as herbal teas and fruit-infused water.

Omega-3 Fatty Acids: Omega-3 fatty acids are important for the baby's brain development. Include fatty fish, walnuts, flaxseeds, and chia seeds in your diet to ensure an adequate intake of these essential fatty acids.

Vitamin D: Breast milk may not provide sufficient vitamin D, so it is important for breastfeeding women to ensure an adequate intake of this vitamin. Good sources of vitamin D include fortified dairy products, fatty fish, and sunlight exposure.

Meal Planning for Nursing Women

Here is an example of a day's meal plan for a nursing woman:

Breakfast: Oatmeal topped with sliced bananas and a drizzle of honey.

Snack: A handful of mixed nuts and dried fruits.

Lunch: Grilled chicken or tofu wrap with mixed greens and avocado.

Snack: Greek yogurt with a sprinkle of granola and fresh berries.

Dinner: Baked salmon with roasted vegetables and quinoa.

Snack: A small bowl of cottage cheese with sliced peaches.

Remember to listen to your body's hunger and fullness cues and adjust portion sizes accordingly. It is also important to continue taking a prenatal vitamin and consult with a healthcare professional for personalized advice.

Conclusion

Maintaining a balanced diet is crucial for the health and well-being of pregnant and nursing women. By focusing on nutrient-dense foods and meeting the increased nutrient requirements, women can support the growth and development of their babies while also taking care of their own nutritional needs. Remember to consult with a healthcare professional for personalized advice and guidance throughout your pregnancy and breastfeeding journey.

Balanced Diet for Older Adults

As we age, our bodies undergo various changes, including changes in metabolism, nutrient absorption, and overall health. It becomes increasingly important for older adults to maintain a balanced diet to support their changing nutritional needs and promote optimal health and well-being. A balanced diet for older adults should focus on providing essential nutrients while also considering any specific health conditions or dietary restrictions. In this section, we will explore the key considerations and recommendations for a balanced diet for older adults.

Nutritional Needs of Older Adults

As we age, our bodies require fewer calories due to a decrease in metabolism and physical activity levels. However, the need for essential nutrients remains the same, if not higher, to support healthy aging and prevent age-related diseases. Here are some key nutrients that older adults should focus on:

Protein: Adequate protein intake is crucial for maintaining muscle mass, strength, and overall health. Older adults should aim for 1-1.2 grams of protein per kilogram of body weight per day. Good sources of protein include lean meats, poultry, fish, eggs, dairy products, legumes, and tofu.

Calcium and Vitamin D: Calcium and vitamin D are essential for maintaining bone health and preventing osteoporosis. Older adults should aim for 1200-1500 milligrams of calcium per day and 800-1000 international units (IU) of vitamin D per day. Good sources of calcium include dairy products, fortified plant-based milk, leafy green vegetables, and fortified cereals. Vitamin D can be obtained through sunlight exposure and fortified foods or supplements.

Fiber: Adequate fiber intake is important for maintaining digestive health and preventing constipation. Older adults should aim for 25-30 grams of fiber per day. Good sources of fiber include whole grains, fruits, vegetables, legumes, and nuts.

Omega-3 Fatty Acids: Omega-3 fatty acids have been shown to have numerous health benefits, including reducing inflammation and supporting heart health. Good sources of omega-3 fatty acids include fatty fish (such as salmon, mackerel, and sardines), flaxseeds, chia seeds, and walnuts.

B Vitamins: B vitamins, including B12, folate, and B6, play a crucial role in energy production, brain function, and the formation of red blood cells. Older adults may have a decreased ability to absorb B12 from food, so it is important to include sources such as fortified cereals, lean meats, fish, and dairy products in their diet.

Key Considerations for a Balanced Diet

In addition to meeting the specific nutritional needs of older adults, there are some key considerations to keep in mind when planning a balanced diet:

Hydration: Older adults may have a decreased sense of thirst, which can put them at risk of dehydration. It is important for older adults to drink an adequate amount of fluids throughout the day, even if they do not feel thirsty. Water, herbal teas, and low-sodium soups are good options for staying hydrated.

Portion Control: As metabolism slows down with age, it is important to practice portion control to avoid overeating and maintain a healthy weight. Older adults should focus on consuming nutrient-dense foods in appropriate portion sizes.

Food Safety: Older adults may have a weakened immune system, making them more susceptible to foodborne illnesses. It is important to practice proper food safety measures, such as washing hands, cooking foods to the appropriate temperature, and avoiding cross-contamination.

Medication Interactions: Some medications can interact with certain nutrients, affecting their absorption or effectiveness. It is important for older adults to consult with their healthcare provider or a registered dietitian to ensure that their diet does not interfere with their medications.

Sample Meal Plan for Older Adults

Here is a sample meal plan that incorporates the key considerations and recommendations for a balanced diet for older adults:

Breakfast: Oatmeal topped with berries and a sprinkle of ground flaxseeds, a boiled egg, and a cup of herbal tea.

Snack: Greek yogurt with a handful of mixed nuts.

Lunch: Grilled chicken breast with steamed vegetables (such as broccoli, carrots, and cauliflower) and a side of quinoa.

Snack: Sliced apple with almond butter.

Dinner: Baked salmon with roasted sweet potatoes and a side salad with mixed greens, cherry tomatoes, and a drizzle of olive oil and balsamic vinegar.

Evening Snack: A small handful of walnuts and a cup of chamomile tea.

Remember, this is just a sample meal plan, and individual nutritional needs may vary. It is important for older adults to listen to their bodies, consult with healthcare professionals, and make adjustments based on their specific needs and preferences.

In conclusion, a balanced diet for older adults should focus on providing adequate nutrients while considering specific nutritional needs and health conditions. By incorporating nutrient-dense foods, practicing portion control, staying hydrated, and considering key considerations, older adults can support healthy aging and overall well-being.

Balanced Diet for Athletes and Active Individuals

Athletes and active individuals have unique nutritional needs due to their increased physical activity levels and higher energy requirements. A balanced diet plays a crucial role in supporting their performance, enhancing recovery, and maintaining overall health. This section will explore the specific dietary considerations for athletes and provide practical tips for optimizing their nutrition.

Energy Requirements for Athletes

Athletes engage in regular physical activity, which significantly increases their energy expenditure.

The energy needs of athletes vary depending on factors such as age, gender, body composition, training intensity, and duration. It is essential for athletes to consume an adequate amount of calories to fuel their workouts and support optimal performance.

To determine their energy requirements, athletes can use formulas like the Harris-Benedict equation or consult with a registered dietitian specializing in sports nutrition. These calculations take into account factors such as basal metabolic rate (BMR) and activity level to estimate the daily calorie needs.

Macronutrient Ratios for Athletes

While the macronutrient ratios for athletes may vary depending on their specific sport or training goals, a general guideline is to consume a balanced ratio of carbohydrates, proteins, and fats.

Carbohydrates are the primary source of energy for athletes, especially during high-intensity activities. They provide readily available fuel for the muscles and help replenish glycogen stores. Athletes should focus on consuming complex carbohydrates such as whole grains, fruits, vegetables, and legumes. These foods provide sustained energy release and essential nutrients.

Proteins are crucial for muscle repair, growth, and recovery. Athletes should aim to consume an adequate amount of high-quality protein sources such as lean meats, poultry, fish, eggs, dairy products, legumes, and plant-based proteins. The recommended protein intake for athletes is generally higher than that of sedentary individuals, ranging from 1.2 to 2.0 grams per kilogram of body weight per day.

Fats play a vital role in providing energy, supporting hormone production, and aiding in the absorption of fat-soluble vitamins. Athletes should focus on consuming healthy fats from sources such as avocados, nuts, seeds, olive oil, and fatty fish. It is important to choose unsaturated fats over saturated and trans fats to promote heart health.

Hydration for Athletes

Proper hydration is crucial for athletes to maintain performance, prevent dehydration, and support recovery. Athletes lose fluids through sweat during exercise, and it is essential to replenish these losses to avoid dehydration.

The American College of Sports Medicine recommends that athletes drink enough fluids to match their sweat losses. This can be estimated by weighing themselves before and after exercise and consuming 16 to 24 ounces of fluid for every pound lost. Water is generally the best choice for hydration, but for intense or prolonged exercise, sports drinks containing electrolytes may be beneficial.

Athletes should also pay attention to their fluid intake throughout the day, not just during exercise.

It is important to drink fluids regularly and listen to their body's thirst cues. Urine color can also be used as a general indicator of hydration status, with lighter urine indicating adequate hydration.

Pre- and Post-Workout Nutrition

Proper nutrition before and after workouts is essential for athletes to optimize performance, support recovery, and prevent muscle breakdown. Pre-workout meals or snacks should provide a combination of carbohydrates and proteins to fuel the workout and enhance muscle glycogen stores.

Examples of pre-workout meals or snacks for athletes include a banana with peanut butter, Greek yogurt with berries, or a turkey and vegetable wrap. It is important to consume these meals or snacks at least one to two hours before exercise to allow for proper digestion.

Post-workout nutrition is crucial for replenishing glycogen stores, repairing muscle tissue, and promoting recovery. Athletes should aim to consume a combination of carbohydrates and proteins within 30 to 60 minutes after exercise. This can be achieved through options such as a protein shake with a banana, a chicken and quinoa salad, or a smoothie with Greek yogurt and fruits.

Nutrient Timing and Supplements

Nutrient timing refers to the strategic timing of nutrient intake to optimize performance and recovery. While the overall nutrient intake throughout the day is crucial, certain nutrients may be more beneficial when consumed before, during, or after exercise.

Carbohydrates consumed before exercise can provide readily available energy, while carbohydrates consumed during prolonged exercise can help maintain blood sugar levels and delay fatigue. Protein consumed after exercise can enhance muscle protein synthesis and aid in recovery.

While a well-balanced diet can generally provide all the necessary nutrients for athletes, certain supplements may be beneficial in specific situations. However, it is important to note that supplements should not replace whole foods and should be used under the guidance of a healthcare professional or registered dietitian.

Examples of commonly used supplements for athletes include protein powders, creatine, branched-chain amino acids (BCAAs), and electrolyte supplements. It is important to remember that supplements should be used to complement a balanced diet and not as a substitute for proper nutrition.

Conclusion

A balanced diet is essential for athletes and active individuals to support their performance, enhance recovery, and maintain overall health. By understanding their energy requirements, optimizing macronutrient ratios, staying hydrated, and paying attention to pre- and post-workout nutrition, athletes can fuel their bodies effectively and achieve their goals. It is important for athletes to consult with a registered dietitian specializing in sports nutrition to develop personalized nutrition plans that meet their specific needs.

SUSTAINABLE EATING

Understanding Sustainable Eating

Sustainable eating is a concept that focuses on making food choices that are not only beneficial for our health but also for the environment. It involves considering the impact of our food production and consumption on the planet and making conscious decisions to minimize harm and promote long-term sustainability. By adopting sustainable eating practices, we can contribute to the preservation of natural resources, reduce greenhouse gas emissions, and support a more resilient and equitable food system.

The Environmental Impact of Food Choices

Our food choices have a significant impact on the environment. The production, processing, transportation, and disposal of food all contribute to various environmental issues. Here are some key aspects to consider:

1. Land Use and Deforestation

The expansion of agriculture to meet the growing demand for food has led to deforestation and habitat destruction. Forests are cleared to make way for croplands and livestock grazing, resulting in the loss of biodiversity and the release of carbon dioxide into the atmosphere. By choosing sustainably produced food, such as organic or locally sourced options, we can help reduce the need for deforestation.

2. Water Usage and Pollution

Agriculture is a major consumer of freshwater resources. Irrigation for crops and water requirements for livestock contribute to water scarcity in many regions. Additionally, the use of fertilizers and pesticides in conventional farming practices can contaminate water sources, leading to pollution and ecosystem degradation. Opting for water-efficient crops and supporting sustainable farming methods can help conserve water and protect water quality.

3. Greenhouse Gas Emissions

The production and transportation of food contribute to greenhouse gas emissions, primarily carbon dioxide, methane, and nitrous oxide. These gases trap heat in the atmosphere, leading to global warming and climate change. Livestock farming, particularly the production of beef and lamb, is a significant source of methane emissions. By reducing our consumption of animal products and choosing plant-based alternatives, we can lower our carbon footprint.

4. Food Waste

Food waste is a significant issue that exacerbates environmental problems. When food is wasted, all the resources used in its production, including water, energy, and land, are also wasted. Additionally, decomposing food in landfills produces methane, a potent greenhouse gas. By practicing mindful consumption, planning meals, and properly storing and utilizing leftovers, we can minimize food waste and its environmental impact.

Tips for Sustainable Food Shopping and Consumption

Making sustainable food choices doesn't have to be complicated. Here are some practical tips to help you incorporate sustainable eating into your daily life:

1. Choose Locally Sourced and Seasonal Foods

Support local farmers and reduce the carbon footprint associated with long-distance transportation by opting for locally sourced foods. Seasonal produce is often fresher, tastier, and requires fewer resources for cultivation. Visit farmers' markets or join a community-supported agriculture (CSA) program to access a variety of locally grown foods.

2. Prioritize Plant-Based Foods

Plant-based diets have been shown to have a lower environmental impact compared to diets rich in animal products. Incorporate more fruits, vegetables, whole grains, legumes, nuts, and seeds into your meals. Experiment with plant-based recipes and explore the wide range of delicious and nutritious plant-based alternatives available today.

3. Reduce Food Waste

Plan your meals, make a shopping list, and buy only what you need. Properly store perishable foods to extend their shelf life. Get creative with using leftovers and consider composting food scraps. By reducing food waste, you not only save money but also contribute to a more sustainable food system.

4. Minimize Packaging Waste

Choose products with minimal packaging or opt for packaging that is recyclable or made from sustainable materials. Consider buying in bulk to reduce packaging waste. Bring your own reusable bags, containers, and water bottles when shopping or dining out to minimize single-use plastic waste.

5. Support Sustainable Farming Practices

Look for organic, fair trade, and Rainforest Alliance certified products. These certifications ensure that the food has been produced using environmentally friendly practices, without the use of harmful chemicals, and with fair treatment of workers. Supporting sustainable farming practices helps protect ecosystems and promotes social responsibility.

6. Reduce Meat and Dairy Consumption

While you don't have to eliminate meat and dairy completely, reducing your consumption can have a significant positive impact on the environment. Consider participating in initiatives like "Meatless Mondays" or try incorporating more plant-based meals into your weekly routine. Choose sustainably sourced and ethically raised animal products when you do consume them.

Promoting Sustainable Eating in Your Community

Individual actions can create a ripple effect and inspire others to adopt sustainable eating practices. Here are some ways you can promote sustainable eating in your community:

1. Share Knowledge and Resources

Educate others about the environmental impact of food choices and the benefits of sustainable eating. Share books, articles, documentaries, and online resources that provide information on sustainable food production and consumption. Encourage discussions and engage in conversations about sustainable eating with friends, family, and colleagues.

2. Support Local Initiatives

Get involved in local food initiatives, such as community gardens, urban farming projects, or food co-ops. Volunteer your time or donate resources to organizations working towards sustainable food systems. By actively participating in these initiatives, you can contribute to the development of a more sustainable and resilient community.

3. Advocate for Policy Changes

Engage with local policymakers and advocate for policies that support sustainable agriculture, reduce food waste, and promote access to healthy and sustainable food options. Write letters, attend public meetings, and join or support organizations that work towards sustainable food policy reform.

4. Teach Sustainable Eating Practices

Organize workshops, cooking classes, or demonstrations to teach others about sustainable eating practices. Share recipes, cooking tips, and meal planning strategies that prioritize sustainable food choices. Encourage schools, community centers, and workplaces to incorporate sustainable eating education into their programs.

5. Lead by Example

Be a role model for sustainable eating by consistently making conscious food choices. Share your experiences, challenges, and successes with others. By leading by example, you can inspire those around you to adopt sustainable eating habits and contribute to a healthier planet.

Remember, sustainable eating is not about perfection but rather progress. Every small step towards making more sustainable food choices can have a positive impact on our health and the environment. Embrace the journey and enjoy the benefits of a balanced diet that nourishes both your body and the planet.

The Environmental Impact of Food Choices

When it comes to making food choices, it's not just about our personal health and well-being. Our food choices also have a significant impact on the environment. The production, transportation, and disposal of food can contribute to various environmental issues such as greenhouse gas emissions, deforestation, water pollution, and loss of biodiversity. In this section, we will explore the environmental impact of our food choices and discuss ways to make more sustainable decisions.

Food Production and Greenhouse Gas Emissions

One of the major contributors to greenhouse gas emissions is the agricultural sector. The production of food, especially meat and dairy products, requires significant amounts of land, water, and energy. Livestock farming, in particular, is responsible for a substantial portion of greenhouse gas emissions, mainly due to methane released by animals and the deforestation associated with creating grazing land and growing animal feed.

To reduce the environmental impact of our food choices, we can consider incorporating more plant-based foods into our diets. Plant-based diets, such as vegetarian or vegan diets, have been shown to have lower greenhouse gas emissions compared to diets that include a high amount of animal products. By reducing our consumption of meat and dairy and opting for plant-based protein sources like legumes, nuts, and tofu, we can significantly reduce our carbon footprint.

Land Use and Deforestation

The expansion of agricultural land to meet the growing demand for food has led to deforestation in many parts of the world. Forests play a crucial role in mitigating climate change by absorbing carbon dioxide from the atmosphere. When forests are cleared for agriculture, the carbon stored in trees is released into the atmosphere, contributing to greenhouse gas emissions.

Choosing food products that are produced sustainably can help reduce deforestation. Look for certifications such as Rainforest Alliance or Forest Stewardship Council (FSC) when purchasing products like coffee, chocolate, or wood-based products. These certifications ensure that the production methods used are environmentally friendly and do not contribute to deforestation.

Water Consumption and Pollution

Water is a precious resource, and the production of food requires significant amounts of water. Agriculture accounts for a large portion of global water consumption, and inefficient irrigation practices can lead to water scarcity and pollution. Additionally, the use of chemical fertilizers and pesticides in agriculture can contaminate water sources, affecting both human and aquatic life.

To minimize water consumption and pollution, we can choose foods that are grown using sustainable farming practices. Organic farming, for example, avoids the use of synthetic fertilizers and pesticides, reducing the risk of water pollution. Additionally, supporting local farmers who practice sustainable irrigation methods can help conserve water resources in your community.

Biodiversity Loss and Genetic Modification

The expansion of agriculture has also led to the loss of biodiversity. Large-scale monoculture farming, where a single crop is grown over vast areas, can deplete the soil of nutrients and increase the risk of pests and diseases. This often leads to the use of chemical pesticides and fertilizers, further impacting the environment.

By diversifying our diets and supporting sustainable farming practices, we can help promote biodiversity. Choosing locally grown and seasonal produce can encourage farmers to cultivate a variety of crops, preserving genetic diversity and reducing the reliance on genetically modified organisms (GMOs). Additionally, supporting organic farming practices can help protect soil health and promote a more sustainable food system.

Food Waste and Packaging

Food waste is a significant environmental issue. When food is wasted, all the resources used in its production, including water, energy, and land, are also wasted. Food waste that ends up in landfills produces methane, a potent greenhouse gas.

To reduce food waste, we can practice mindful shopping and meal planning. By planning our meals, we can buy only what we need and use leftovers creatively. Additionally, choosing products with minimal packaging or opting for reusable containers can help reduce the amount of waste generated from our food choices.

Conclusion

Our food choices have a profound impact on the environment. By considering the environmental implications of our food production and consumption, we can make more sustainable choices that benefit both our health and the planet. From reducing our meat and dairy consumption to supporting sustainable farming practices and minimizing food waste, every small change we make can contribute to a more sustainable food system. Let's strive to create a balanced diet that not only nourishes our bodies but also supports a healthier planet for future generations.

Tips for Sustainable Food Shopping and Consumption

Sustainable food shopping and consumption are essential aspects of adopting a balanced diet. By making conscious choices about the food we buy and consume, we can contribute to a healthier planet and support sustainable agricultural practices. In this section, we will explore some practical tips for sustainable food shopping and consumption.

1. Choose Locally Sourced Foods

One of the most effective ways to reduce the carbon footprint of your food is to choose locally sourced options. Locally produced foods require less transportation, which means fewer greenhouse gas emissions. Additionally, supporting local farmers and producers helps to strengthen the local economy and promotes sustainable farming practices. Look for farmers' markets, community-supported agriculture (CSA) programs, and local food co-ops to find fresh, locally sourced produce, dairy products, and meats.

2. Opt for Organic and Sustainable Certification

When shopping for food, look for organic and sustainable certifications. Organic foods are grown without the use of synthetic pesticides, herbicides, and genetically modified organisms (GMOs). By choosing organic options, you support farming practices that prioritize soil health, biodiversity, and the reduction of chemical inputs. Similarly, sustainable certifications, such as the Marine Stewardship Council (MSC) for seafood or the Rainforest Alliance for coffee and cocoa, ensure that the products are sourced from environmentally responsible and socially equitable practices.

3. Reduce Food Waste

Food waste is a significant issue that contributes to environmental degradation. By reducing food waste, we can minimize the resources used in food production and decrease methane emissions from landfills. Plan your meals and create a shopping list to avoid buying more than you need. Properly store perishable items to extend their shelf life, and repurpose leftovers into new meals. Composting is another great way to divert food waste from landfills and create nutrient-rich soil for your garden.

4. Embrace Seasonal Eating

Choosing seasonal produce not only supports local farmers but also reduces the energy required for transportation and storage. Seasonal fruits and vegetables are often fresher, tastier, and more nutritious. Additionally, by embracing seasonal eating, you can enjoy a diverse range of flavors throughout the year. Consider exploring farmers' markets or joining a CSA to discover the abundance of seasonal produce available in your area.

5. Minimize Packaging Waste

Packaging waste is a significant contributor to environmental pollution. When shopping, opt for products with minimal packaging or choose items with eco-friendly packaging materials. Buying in bulk can also help reduce packaging waste. Bring your own reusable bags, produce bags, and containers to the grocery store or farmers' market to further minimize single-use plastic waste.

6. Support Sustainable Seafood Choices

Overfishing and destructive fishing practices have led to the depletion of many marine species and the degradation of marine ecosystems. When purchasing seafood, look for sustainable options certified by organizations like the MSC or the Aquaculture Stewardship Council (ASC). These certifications ensure that the seafood is sourced from well-managed fisheries or responsible aquaculture operations.

7. Reduce Meat Consumption

The production of meat, especially beef, has a significant environmental impact due to deforestation, water usage, and greenhouse gas emissions. Consider reducing your meat consumption by incorporating more plant-based meals into your diet. Plant-based proteins like legumes, tofu, and tempeh are not only environmentally friendly but also provide essential nutrients. If you choose to eat meat, opt for sustainably raised and locally sourced options.

8. Grow Your Own Food

If you have the space and resources, consider growing your own food. Gardening allows you to have control over the cultivation process, ensuring that your produce is free from harmful chemicals. It also reduces the need for transportation and packaging. Even if you have limited space, you can grow herbs, salad greens, or tomatoes in containers on a balcony or windowsill.

9. Support Fair Trade Products

Fair trade products ensure that farmers and workers receive fair wages and work in safe conditions. When purchasing coffee, tea, chocolate, or other imported goods, look for fair trade certifications. By supporting fair trade, you contribute to the well-being of farmers and promote sustainable farming practices.

10. Educate Yourself and Spread Awareness

Continuing to educate yourself about sustainable food practices is crucial for making informed choices. Stay updated on current issues related to food sustainability, such as climate change, food waste, and agricultural practices. Share your knowledge with friends, family, and your community to inspire others to adopt sustainable food shopping and consumption habits.

By implementing these tips for sustainable food shopping and consumption, you can make a positive impact on both your health and the health of the planet. Remember, small changes in our daily habits can collectively create a significant difference in building a more sustainable future.

Promoting Sustainable Eating in Your Community

Sustainable eating is not just about making conscious choices for your own health and the environment, but also about spreading awareness and inspiring others to do the same. By promoting sustainable eating in your community, you can contribute to a healthier planet and encourage others to make positive changes in their dietary habits. Here are some effective ways to promote sustainable eating in your community:

1. Organize Community Events and Workshops

One of the best ways to promote sustainable eating is by organizing community events and workshops. These events can include cooking demonstrations, educational talks, and interactive sessions where participants can learn about the benefits of sustainable eating and how to incorporate it into their daily lives. Invite local chefs, nutritionists, and environmental experts to share their knowledge and expertise. Encourage participants to ask questions and engage in discussions to foster a sense of community and shared learning.

2. Collaborate with Local Farmers and Food Suppliers

Supporting local farmers and food suppliers is an essential aspect of sustainable eating. Reach out to local farmers' markets, community-supported agriculture (CSA) programs, and organic food cooperatives to establish partnerships. Collaborate with them to organize farm visits, where community members can learn about sustainable farming practices and the importance of buying locally grown produce. Encourage community members to support these local businesses by purchasing their products and incorporating them into their meals.

3. Start a Community Garden

A community garden is a fantastic way to promote sustainable eating and foster a sense of community. Identify a suitable location and gather interested individuals to start a garden together. Encourage participants to grow their own fruits, vegetables, and herbs using organic and sustainable gardening practices. Organize regular gardening workshops and share tips on composting, natural pest control, and water conservation. The produce from the community garden can be shared among participants or donated to local food banks, further promoting sustainable eating within the community.

4. Share Sustainable Recipes and Meal Ideas

Food is a powerful tool for inspiring change. Create a platform, such as a community website or social media group, where members can share sustainable recipes and meal ideas. Encourage participants to use locally sourced, seasonal ingredients and reduce food waste. Share tips on meal planning, batch cooking, and creative ways to use leftovers. By sharing delicious and sustainable recipes, you can inspire others to make conscious choices in their own kitchens.

5. Engage with Local Schools and Educational Institutions

Children and young adults are the future of our communities. Engage with local schools and educational institutions to promote sustainable eating among students. Offer to conduct workshops or give presentations on the importance of sustainable eating and its impact on the environment. Collaborate with school cafeterias to introduce more sustainable and plant-based options in their menus. Encourage the establishment of school gardens where students can learn about growing their own food and the principles of sustainable agriculture.

6. Advocate for Sustainable Food Policies

Get involved in local government and advocate for sustainable food policies. Attend town hall meetings, write letters to local representatives, and join community organizations that focus on sustainable living. Push for initiatives such as supporting local farmers, reducing food waste, and promoting plant-based options in public institutions. By actively participating in the decision-making process, you can help shape a more sustainable food system in your community.

7. Host Film Screenings and Discussion Panels

Film screenings and discussion panels are effective ways to raise awareness about sustainable eating. Choose documentaries and films that highlight the environmental impact of our food choices and the benefits of sustainable eating. After the screening, host a discussion panel with local experts to delve deeper into the topics presented in the film. Encourage participants to share their thoughts, ask questions, and brainstorm ideas for promoting sustainable eating within the community.

8. Support Local Food Recovery Programs

Food waste is a significant issue that contributes to environmental degradation. Support local food recovery programs that aim to reduce food waste and redistribute surplus food to those in need. Volunteer your time or donate resources to organizations that collect excess food from restaurants, grocery stores, and farms, and distribute it to community members facing food insecurity. By supporting these programs, you not only promote sustainable eating but also help address social issues within your community.

9. Be a Role Model and Share Your Journey

Lead by example and share your own sustainable eating journey with others. Talk about the positive changes you have made in your diet and lifestyle and how they have benefited you and the environment. Share your challenges, successes, and tips for incorporating sustainable eating into everyday life. By being open and transparent about your experiences, you can inspire others to embark on their own sustainable eating journeys.

10. Foster a Supportive and Inclusive Community

Creating a supportive and inclusive community is crucial for promoting sustainable eating. Encourage open dialogue, respect different dietary choices, and provide a safe space for individuals to ask questions and seek guidance. Foster a sense of belonging and support among community members, as sustainable eating is a journey that requires ongoing learning and adaptation. By creating a positive and inclusive environment, you can empower individuals to make sustainable choices and contribute to a healthier and more sustainable community.

Remember, promoting sustainable eating in your community is a collective effort. By taking these steps and encouraging others to join you, you can make a significant impact on the health of both individuals and the planet. Start small, be persistent, and celebrate every positive change made within your community. Together, we can create a more sustainable future through our dietary choices.

References:

Dietary Guidelines for Americans - U.S. Department of Agriculture and U.S. Department of Health and Human Services

The Complete Guide to Sports Nutrition - Anita Bean

Nutrition: Concepts and Controversies - Frances Sizer and Ellie Whitney

The Blue Zones Solution: Eating and Living Like the World's Healthiest People - Dan Buettner

The Plant-Based Solution: America's Healthy Heart Doc's Plan to Power Your Health - Joel K. Kahn, MD

ABOUT THE AUTHOR

Ifeanyichukwu Ezekwem

Ifeanyichukwu Ezekwem is a debut author and a dedicated pharmacist with a passion for promoting health and well-being.

Combining their expertise in pharmacy with their love for educating, Ifeanyichukwu Ezekwem simplifies the complexities of nutrition in a way that's accessible to everyone. This debut work showcases their commitment to sharing knowledge and improving lives through the power of words.

When not writing, Ifeanyichukwu Ezekwem continues to make a positive impact in the world of healthcare, and helping individuals lead healthier lives. "Basics of Balanced Diet" is just the beginning of what promises to be an exciting literary journey for this talented author.